Manual of

ADVANCED PREHOSPITAL CARE

2nd Edition

Robert J. Brady Co.
A Prentice-Hall Publishing and Communications Company
Bowie, Maryland

Executive Editor: Richard A. Weimer
Art Director: Don Sellers
Index: Leah Kramer

We wish to acknowledge the contribution of Josie Harding, RN, our co-author of the first edition.

Manual of Advanced Prehospital Care, 2nd Edition

Library of Congress Cataloging in Publication Data

Walraven, Gail, 1949-
    Manual of advanced prehospital care.

    Second ed. of: Manual of advanced prehospital care /
authors, Gail Walraven . . . [et al.]. c1978.
      Bibliography: p.
      Includes index.
      1. Medical emergencies—Handbooks, manuals, etc.
2. Drugs—Handbooks, manuals, etc. 3. Arrhythmia—
Handbooks, manuals, etc. I. Manual of advanced
prehospital care. [DNLM: 1. Allied health personnel—
Handbooks. 2. Emergency medical services—
Handbooks. WX 215 W221m]
RC86.7.W357   1983   616'.025   83-2580
ISBN 0-89303-252-2

Prentice-Hall International, Inc., London
Prentice-Hall Canada, Inc., Scarborough, Ontario
Prentice-Hall of Australia, Pty., Ltd., Sydney
Prentice-Hall of India Private Limited, New Delhi
Prentice-Hall of Japan, Inc., Tokyo
Prentice-Hall of Southeast Asia Pte. Ltd., Singapore
Whitehall Books, Limited, Petone, New Zealand
Editora Prentice-Hall Do Brasil LTDA., Rio de Janeiro

Printed in the United States of America

83 84 85 86 87 88 89 90 91 92 93   10 9 8 7 6 5 4 3 2 1

CONTENTS

SECTION I: MEDICAL MANAGEMENT

CONTENTS

Chronic Obstructive Pulmonary Disease
Cold Injuries
Coma of Unknown Origin
Diabetes
Diving Accidents
Drowning (Near)
Heat Exposure
Hypertensive Crisis
Hyperventilation Syndrome
Neurological Trauma
Obstetrical Emergencies
Overdose
Poisoning
Pulmonary Edema
Radiation Exposure
Rape and Sexual Assault
Seizures
Shock (Hypovolemic)
Smoke/Gas Inhalation
Trauma (Multi-System)
Venomous Land Animals
Venomous Water Animals

INTRODUCTION

This section on Medical Management lists alphabetically virtually all of the acute medical conditions which the paramedic can expect to find in a prehospital setting. A short narrative profiles each of these conditions, including brief pathophysiology, signs and symptoms, and necessary field treatment. Each profile is followed by a concise Treatment Protocol for field management of the condition.

The Treatment Protocols are designed to be a summary of all the important facts about a particular problem. They are *not* intended to dictate medical practice. In this format, the protocols can be modified to conform to local medical practices. These protocols are not a substitute for your own medical knowledge, experience, and judgement; you should make your own decisions based on individual patient situations.

As with other sections of *Manual of Advanced Prehospital Care,* this section does not attempt to teach, but does gather summary information into a clear synopsis of pertinent material. To use this section, first read the profiles as they exist. Then go back and modify each one if necessary to coincide with the teachings and policies of your local program. Check with your instructors, medical advisors, and other resources to be certain your changes are accurate. Once these modifications are complete you can use the section as a basis for study. To assess your retention and understanding of the material, complete the Self-Assessment Questions at the end of the section.

ABDOMINAL PAIN
(Nontraumatic)

A wide variety of medical conditions can cause severe abdominal pain, or abdominal pain of such sudden onset that emergency aid is requested. Included in these disorders are appendicitis, ulcers, herniation, pelvic inflammatory disease, dissecting abdominal aneurysm, cholelithiasis, renal calculi, ruptured ovarian cyst, ectopic pregnancy, and virtually countless others.

The clinical picture of abdominal pain is usually one of guarding, possibly with the knees drawn up toward the chest and the arms protecting the abdomen. The patient may be nauseated or may have vomited. There may be a history of either constipation or diarrhea, and/or obvious abdominal distension. Additionally, each of the possible clinical causes of the pain can have its own characteristic picture, such as the anxiety and knife-like tearing pain of the dissection aneurysm.

Because of the great variety of possible causes of abdominal pain and the intensive diagnostic and laboratory tools that are required for an accurate identification of the source of the pain, the primary emphasis of field management is supportive. Assessment should include attention to ABCs, vital signs, a pertinent medical history, and a complete physical exam.

Don't palpate the abdomen extensively. A hand placed gently on the abdomen can detect rigidity, suggesting internal bleeding. However, extensive palpation is of little value either to the patient or the paramedic. Regardless of the findings, treatment will depend on other clinical signs such as those related to shock, and will not be altered by the results of an extensive examination of the abdomen. More importantly, sophisticated palpation or auscultation of the abdomen will delay transportation and expose the patient to further discomfort.

Field treatment of acute abdominal pain is limited to oxygen, close monitoring of vital signs and an IV of Lactated Ringer's or Normal Saline as a life line. Be aware of the threat of shock, anticipate the signs, and recognize them when they appear. Don't give any food or fluids by mouth, and consider inserting a nasogastric (NG) tube to decompress the stomach. If the patient vomits, urinates or defecates, save a specimen for the hospital. Avoid giving pain medications as they will mask symptoms and interfere with the physician's assessment. Throughout the management of the run move quickly and expeditiously to transport the patient without undue delay.

TREATMENT PROTOCOL: ABDOMINAL PAIN (NONTRAUMATIC)

History

- What precipitated the pain?
- What type of pain is it?
- Where is the pain located?
- Does the pain radiate?
- Has the patient ever had it before?
- What is the severity of the pain?
- When did it start?
- What is the pain associated with?
- Has the patient had any recent illnesses or operations?
- Did the patient suffer recent trauma?
- Has the patient had any changes in bowel or bladder habits?
- Has the patient been nauseated or vomited?
- Did the patient ingest any unusual substances?
- Has there been any vaginal bleeding or discharge?
- Is there any possibility of pregnancy?

Physical Exam

- What is the respiratory rate, rhythm and effectiveness?
- What is the patient's level of consciousness?
- What is the skin color, moisture, and temperature?
- What are the vital signs?
- What is the EKG pattern?
- Are there any signs of dehydration?
- Is the patient febrile?
- Is the patient "guarding?"
- Is there bruising, a pulsating mass; scars on the abdomen?
- Is the abdomen rigid? Distended?

Differential Diagnosis

- appendicitis
- ulcers

- herniation
- pelvic inflammatory disease
- ectopic pregnancy
- cholelithiasis
- renal calculi
- myocardial infarction
- dissecting abdominal aneurysm
- ruptured ovarian cyst
- poisoning
- overdose

Treatment

1. Ensure airway patency, give oxygen and ventilate if necessary.
2. Start an IV of Lactated Ringer's or Normal Saline TKO; if hypovolemic shock is suspected run at a rate to maintain blood pressure.
3. Apply antishock trousers; inflate if necessary.
4. Consider an NG tube.
5. Do not give analgesics or oral fluids.
6. Do not waste time palpating the the abdomen extensively or eliciting bowel sounds.

Special Note

- Save a sample of any stool, urine or emesis an͏ hospital for analysis.

Pediatric Note

- In a child, suspect poisoning.

Transport

- Patient should be transpo͏
- Do not delay transportation

ABDOMINAL TRAUMA

Traumatic injuries to the abdomen can be blunt (e.g., being struck in the abdomen), or penetrating (e.g., a gunshot or knife wound).

Blunt trauma can be deceiving because there may not be bruises on the skin, and internal damage can be far worse than external appearance suggests. Blunt abdominal trauma frequently causes damage to the spleen or liver, resulting in internal hemorrhage, and a patient with no outward signs of trauma can quickly become cool, clammy, diaphoretic, pale, confused, and unconscious.

Vital signs may be within normal limits initially and then change to tachycardia, tachypnea, and hypotension as internal blood loss increases. Orthostatic vital signs may confirm any suspicion of hypovolemia. On secondary survey, check specifically for abdominal distention, bruising, tenderness, rigidity, and/or guarding.

Penetrating trauma is similar to blunt trauma in that it can also cause hemorrhagic shock and greater internal damage than appears on the body surface. In penetrating trauma you must also evaluate entry and exit wounds as well as external blood loss.

If a knife or similar instrument is protruding, do not remove it, but stabilize it in place while controlling external hemorrhage with direct pressure. An impaled object may be removed as a last resort if it becomes necessary to inflate the abdominal section of the antishock trousers. Depending on the length of the penetrating object and the angle of insertion, the thoracic cavity may also be involved, and the patient might suffer respiratory compromise.

Specific field treatment of abdominal trauma includes high-flow oxygen, monitoring of EKG, IV NS or RL to maintain blood pressure, control of ernal hemorrhage, and antishock trousers. If evisceration is present r with a saline-soaked dressing and do not attmept to push the protru- back in. Transport the patient promptly and do not give any pain ation or oral fluids.

TREATMENT PROTOCOL:
ABDOMINAL TRAUMA

as the mechanism of injury?
the injury?

- What is the estimated blood loss?
- Is there any pain?
- Was the trauma blunt or penetrating?
- What was the time of injury?
- When was the onset of symptoms?

Physical Exam

- What is the respiratory rate, rhythm, and effectiveness?
- What is the level of consciousness?
- What is the skin color, temperature, and moisture?
- What are the vital signs?
- What are the lung sounds?
- Are there any apparent injuries on front or back?
- Is the abdomen rigid, distended, tender, or bruised?
- Are there any associated injuries?
- Are there any penetrating objects?
- If gunshot or knife injury, are there entry or exit wounds?

Differential Diagnosis

- Perform thorough exam for other injuries.

Treatment

1. Ensure airway patency, give oxygen and ventilate if necessary.
2. Control bleeding
3. Start an IV or RL or NS and run at a rate to maintain blood pressure.
4. If blood loss is significant, antishock trousers might be indicated.
5. Immobilize penetrating objects, but do not remove unless antishock trousers must be inflated over the area.
6. If the patient has an eviscerated bowel, cover with saline-soaked pads.
7. Do not give analgesics or oral fluids.
8. Do not waste time palpating the abdomen extensively or eliciting bowel sounds.

Special Note

- Any high abdominal injury should be suspected of involving the thoracic cavity.

Pediatric Note

- Consider child abuse.

Transport

- Immobilize patient before moving, if indicated.
- Transport the patient as soon as possible.

AIRWAY OBSTRUCTION

An airway obstruction is anything which interferes with the intake of air into the lungs. The two major causes of airway obstruction are foreign bodies and edema. Types of foreign bodies include the tongue, food, dentures, emesis, blood, broken teeth, and miscellaneous objects which get lodged in the upper airway. Edema in the posterior pharynx or the larynx can also cause airway obstruction. This is most commonly seen in respiratory burns, allergic reaction/anaphylaxis, and pediatric diseases such as croup and epiglottitis.

Airway obstruction can be either partial or complete, depending on the degree to which air exchange is obstructed. A *partial obstruction* can cause decreased oxygen intake, followed by arrhythmias, seizures, and other signs of hypoxia. Signs of a partial obstruction include respiratory stridor, crowing, use of accessory muscles such as sternal retraction and intercostal indrawing, restlessness, and fatigue. The patient may have a hoarse voice, severe anxiety, and a cough. A *complete* obstruction causes anoxia which leads to anaerobic metabolism, lactic acidosis, coma, and death. Signs that the obstruction is complete include inability to talk or cough, cyanosis, and desperate clutching at the throat. Unless promptly relieved, unconsciousness, seizures, and cardiac arrest will follow quickly.

Treatment of Foreign Body Obstruction

Foreign body obstruction occurs most frequently during meals (especially if alcohol is ingested), in children, in unconscious patients, and in traumatic situations. If the person is still conscious and coughing, suspect a partial obstruction and treat cautiously. Encourage coughing, give oxygen and emotional support, and transport rapidly. Avoid performing manual maneuvers, as they might turn a partial obstruction into a complete one.

Treatment of a total obstruction caused by a foreign body in the upper airway depends on whether or not the patient is conscious and attempting to clear his/her own airway. If so, a series of back blows and manual thrusts is often successful in dislodging the foreign object. If the patient is unconscious, or becomes unconscious, use a laryngoscope to visualize the offending object and remove or deflect it with the Magill forceps. If these techniques are not immediately successful, a repetitive series of backblows, manual thrusts, mechanical removal with Magill forceps, and ventilation attempts can be repeated enroute to the hospital. Some systems train their personnel to perform a cricothyrotomy to create a patent airway below the site of obstruction. This should only be done after more conventional methods have failed, and only if your system prepares and authorizes you to perform it.

Treatment of Laryngeal Edema

Edema of the mucous membranes is the most likely cause of airway obstruction following respiratory burns or during an allergic reaction. Partial obstruction should be treated with high-flow oxygen, reassurance, and rapid transport. Start an IV TKO for possible drug and/or fluid administration. Total obstruction is treated with endotracheal intubation and assisted ventilation, or if authorized, cricothyrotomy. If the edema is a direct result of allergic reaction, epinephrine might be effective in counteracting the swelling. As with any hypoxic patient, give high-concentration oxygen, monitor EKG, and transport promptly.

Pediatric Laryngeal Edema

The two most common pediatric disorders which present with symptoms of airway obstruction due to edema are croup and epiglottitis. These disorders are quite similar clinically, and are often difficult to differentiate in the field. *Croup* is caused by a virus, and results in edema of the subglottic tissues. It very rarely progresses to total obstruction. The child usually exhibits a barking cough, inspiratory stridor, and dyspnea which is aided by cool mist. *Epiglottitis* is a bacterial inflammation of the epiglottis. It is extremely dangerous because it can rapidly cause total occlusion of the airway. The signs of epiglottitis include sudden onset of inspiratory stridor, dysphagia, drooling, fever, and extreme anxiety. The chin is often thrust forward in a characteristic posture to facilitate air exchange.

Field treatment of both croup and epiglottitis is primarily supportive, and includes airway maintenance, high-flow oxygen, and prompt transport. It is extremely important to avoid attempts to visualize the epiglottis since stimulation can cause total obstruction if epiglottitis is present. Should the airway become completely obstructed, attempt to ventilate, insert an endotracheal tube, or perform a cricothyrotomy if authorized.

TREATMENT PROTOCOL: AIRWAY OBSTRUCTION

History

- When did this happen?
- What precipitated the event?
- Was patient eating, vomiting, or putting things in his/her mouth?
- Has patient had a fever or cough?
- Was patient stung by a bee or exposed to an allergen?

Physical Exam

- Is patient exchanging air effectively?
- What are the sounds of respiration?
- What is the level of consciousness?
- Is the patient able to talk or cough?
- What is the skin color?
- Is there any trauma to oropharynx, mandible, or maxilla?
- Is there any sternal retraction, nostril flaring, or intercostal indrawing?
- Is there any soot around mouth, singed nasal hairs, or facial burns?
- What are the vital signs?
- What is the EKG pattern?

Differential Diagnosis

- Differentiate between obstruction due to a foreign body and obstruction due to laryngeal edema.
- Determine whether the obstruction is partial or complete.

Treatment

When Obstruction Is Due to a Foreign Body in the Upper Airway

- If patient is conscious and able to talk or cough:
  1. Leave him/her alone.
  2. Give reassurance.
  3. Encourage him/her to cough.
  4. Give oxygen if patient will tolerate it.
- If the patient is conscious but unable to talk or exchange air:
  1. Administer four back blows.
  2. Administer four manual thrusts.
  3. If necessary, repeat steps 1 and 2.
- If patient is unconscious when found or loses consciousness:
  1. Open airway and attempt to ventilate.
  2. Apply four back blows in rapid succession.
  3. Apply four manual thrusts.
  4. Apply the finger sweep.
  5. Reposition the head, open the airway, and attempt to ventilate.
  6. If necessary, repeat steps 2–5.
  7. If the foreign body is directly visible with a laryngoscope, attempt to remove it with Magill forceps.
  8. Consider cricothyrotomy if all other maneuvers fail.

When Obstruction Is Due to Laryngeal Edema

- If allergic reaction is suspected:
  1. Give high-flow oxygen; intubate and assist ventilations if necessary.
  2. Start an IV of 5% D/W TKO.
  3. Follow specific treatment outlined in Allergic Reaction Protocol.
- If Respiratory Burns are suspected:
  1. Remove patient from harmful environment.
  2. Ensure patent airway (intubate if necessary); assist ventilations if necessary.
  3. Administer 100% oxygen.

4. Start an IV of 5% D/W TKO; may use RL or NS if volume replacement is needed.

5. If bronchospasm is present, may give Aminophylline 3–6 mg/kg in at least 20 ml 5% D/W IV Volutrol over a minimum of 20 minutes.

- If Croup/Epiglottitis is suspected:

1. Ensure patent airway, intubate if necessary.

2. Administer high-flow oxygen; assist ventilations if necessary.

3. Avoid visualizing epiglottitis, since to do so may cause complete obstruction.

4. If all other measures fail and you are authorized, consider performing a cricothyrotomy.

Special Note

- Once obstruction is relieved, assess patient for bilateral air movement, color, respiratory effort, and vital signs; monitor EKG, give high-flow oxygen, and start an IV of 5% D/W TKO if indicated.
- All patients in this category must be evaluated at the hospital.
- If patient goes into cardiac arrest, re-establishing the airway is still the main priority of treatment.

Pediatric Note

- Children often insert foreign objects into nose or mouth.
- Abdominal thrusts are not recommended for infants and small children.
- Aminophylline should be used cautiously in children under age 12.

Transport

- No need for "red lights and siren" transport if patient is stabilized.

ALLERGIC REACTION / ANAPHYLAXIS

In a simple allergic reaction, the body reacts to a foreign substance, or antigen, by releasing histamine. This causes the characteristic rash, redness, swelling, and itching of allergy. Anaphylaxis is a severe allergic reaction, usually to an insect sting or a medication. In anaphylaxis, the release of histamine is more profound, causing the bronchial tree to go into spasm. Histamine also dilates the peripheral vessels and alters permeability of cell membranes, allowing escape of fluid volume into the tissue spaces.

Acute anaphylaxis is usually an immediate response, but may be delayed from 10 to 30 minutes. The symptoms include sudden anxiety and restlessness, often with a pounding or throbbing headache. This is followed by a feeling of suffocation, tightness in the chest, coughing, wheezing, or stridor, and can progress very quickly to total airway obstruction, and profound hypotension. If treatment is not initiated promptly, death or permanent brain damage can result.

The following steps can be taken in the field to treat allergic reaction. First, establish an airway, give oxygen, and evaluate cardiorespiratory status. As rapidly as possible, administer 0.3 mg epinephrine 1:1,000 SC. Epinephrine is a drug with both alpha and beta properties; therefore, it acts to dilate the bronchial tree and constrict the vascular system when given in the recommended dose. Establish an IV of 5% D/W TKO in the event you need to give additional medications. Monitor vital signs and EKG frequently to determine effectiveness of therapy.

Following the administration of epinephrine, Benadryl can be given to prevent further reaction by blocking histamine from the receptor sites. If the toxin was introduced through the skin, i.e., a bee sting or an injection, you might also administer 0.1 mg epinephrine 1,1000 SC at the site of the reaction (if not a finger or toe) and/or use a constricting band proximal to the site if on an extremity. Both steps decrease the spread of toxin via the circulatory system.

In a severe reaction, additional drug therapy such as IV epinephrine, dopamine, or Aminophylline may be required. Transport the patient with oxygen and pay close attention to vital signs.

TREATMENT PROTOCOL: ALLERGIC REACTION ANAPHYLAXIS

History

- Was patient recently exposed to foods, drugs, insects, or other allergens that may have induced reaction?
- When was patient exposed?

- When did symptoms appear?
- Has the patient had previous allergic reactions?

Physical Exam

- Are there any signs of respiratory distress or tightness in the chest?
- Are there any signs of systemic allergic reaction such as rash, itching, hives, or general swelling?
- What is the level of consciousness?
- What is the skin color, temperature, and moisture?
- What are the vital signs?
- What are the lung sounds?
- What is the EKG pattern?
- Is the patient wearing a Medic-Alert tag?

Differential Diagnosis

- Might be confused with asthma or foreign body obstruction of the upper airway.
- Determine source of the reaction, such as bee, drug, or food.

Treatment

1. Ensure patent airway; intubate and ventilate if necessary.
2. Give high-flow oxygen.
3. Place a constricting band 1 inch proximal to site if feasible.
4. Start an IV of 5% D/W TKO if necessary.
5. Give epinephrine 0.3 mg 1:1,000 SC, may repeat 3 times at 5-min intervals; can also give 0.1 mg 1:1,000 at site if other than fingers or toes; *or,* If laryngeal edema or hypotension is present, give 0.1–0.5 mg epinephrine 1:10,000 IV push; may repeat in 10 min. (not to exceed 0.5 mg in 10 min.)
6. Give Benadryl 25–50 mg slow IV push or deep IM.
7. Keep patient calm; discourage activity.
8. May need additional drug therapy such as Aminophylline, dopamine, or vasopressors.

9. If cardiovascular collapse continues despite drug therapy, apply antishock trousers.
10. May need cricothyrotomy if patient does not respond to drugs and airway becomes totally obstructed.

Special Note

- If reaction is severe, attempt to intubate before edema occludes airway.

Pediatric Note

- Pediatric doses:

  Epinephrine: 0.01 ml/kg (1:1,000) SC; may repeat 3 times at 20 min intervals to a maximum of 0.3 mg; *or* if reaction is severe, 0.01 mg/kg (1:10,000) IV push; may repeat in 10 min (not to exceed 0.5 mg in 10 min).

  Benadryl: 2 mg/kg slow IV push or deep IM

Transport

- May need epinephrine enroute.
- Need not be "red lights and siren" if patient is stabilized.

ARRHYTHMIAS

Cardiac arrhythmias are disturbances in the heart's electrical function. These in turn can cause mechanical malfunctions, and can eventually compromise overall cardiac output. As part of the body's central life support system, cardiac arrhythmias are common to many pathologic states, including cardiac disease, respiratory distress, fluid/electrolyte imbalances, neurological disorders, chemical and metabolic abnormalities, and trauma. They are most predictably linked to myocardial infarction, and are the major cause of death in these patients.

Any patient with the potential for rhythm disturbances should be monitored and receive an IV of 5% D/W TKO as a precaution. If arrhythmias do occur, it is important to remember that the EKG can only provide information about the electrical function of the heart. It is imperative that perfusion parameters such as pulse and blood pressure be monitored concurrently to determine mechanical function.

Three categories of arrhythmias are known to produce symptoms:

Tachycardias:	Heart rate is so fast that ventricular filling time is inadequate; cardiac output drops as stroke volume falls.
Bradycardias:	Heart rate is so slow that it can't maintain an adequate cardiac output.
Ventricular Irritability:	The erratic ventricular contraction isn't effective enough to maintain stroke volume, thus reducing cardiac output.

Each of these mechanisms causes symptoms by reducing cardiac output. Signs of a drop in cardiac output include hypotension, shortness of breath, chest pain, diaphoresis, cool clammy skin, cyanosis, dizziness, and decreasing level of consciousness. Arrhythmias are only treated if they cause, or have the potential to cause signs/symptoms of decreased cardiac output. If the patient is symptomatic measures should be taken to convert the causative rhythm disturbance to a more viable rhythm.

Treatment

Treatment coincides with the major categories of arrhythmias that are known to produce symptoms: bradycardias, tachycardias, and ventricular irritability. *Bradycardias* are treated by enhancing the pacemaker and/or stimulating a higher pacemaker site. Atropine, Isuprel, and Epinephrine are all useful in increasing heart rate. If mechanical malfunction is also suspected, calcium chloride is indicated. Treatment of *tachycardias* is aimed at suppressing the irritable pacemaker by a) stimulating the vagus nerve (with Valsalva's maneuver or carotid sinus massage); or b) drugs that slow impulse formation and/or conduction (such as Digitalis or Inderal); or c) cardioverting to eliminate the irritable focus and allow a normal pacemaker to resume function. *Ventricular irritability* is treated by suppressing the irritable focus with Lidocaine if the patient is still perfusing. If perfusion is compromised, cardioversion or defibrillation can be used to override the irritable site. Irritability associated with recurrent or refractory ventricular fibrillation might require Bretylium to restore a viable rhythm.

In addition to specific arrhythmia treatment, patients with compromised cardiac output often require other resuscitative measures such as CPR, ventilation, and sodium bicarbonate.

TREATMENT PROTOCOL: ARRHYTHMIAS

History

- What is the patient's chief complaint?
- What precipitated symptoms?
- Has the patient ever had this problem before?
- How bad is the problem?
- When did symptoms begin?
- Has the patient ever had cardiac problems or arrhythmias before?
- Is the patient taking any medications?
- What is the past medical history?

Physical Exam

- What is the respiratory rate, rhythm and effectiveness?
- Does the patient show signs of decreased cardiac output?
- What are the vital signs?
- What is the EKG pattern?
- What is the level of consciousness?
- What are the lung sounds?
- What is the skin color, temperature, and moisture?
- Does the patient have distended neck veins or peripheral edema?

Differential Diagnosis

Drop in cardiac output can be caused by
- Tachycardias
- Bradycardias
- Ventricular Irritability

Treatment

Supraventricular Tachyarrhythmias

1. Perform vagotonic maneuvers (Valsalva's maneuver, CSM).

2. Give Inderal, up to 1 mg slow IV push every 5 minutes, for a total of no more than 5 mg, *or* give Digoxin 0.5–0.75 mg per 45 kg (100 lbs) IV push.

3. Perform synchronized cardioversion; if necessary, sedate patient with Valium in increments of 2.5 mg IV push over one minute, up to a total of 20 mg, titrated to effect, *or* 5–10 mg IM.

Supraventricular Bradyarrhythmias

1. Give atropine 0.5 mg IV push; repeat as needed every 5 minutes up to 2 mg.

2. If bradycardia does not respond to atropine, consider Isuprel 2–20 mcg/minute IV drip.

Ventricular Tachyarrhythmias

- *For* PVCs or *ventricular tachycardia* where the patient *is perfusing:*
  1. Give Lidocaine 1 mg/kg slow IV push.
  2. Follow immediately with an IV drip of Lidocaine 2–4 mg/min, *or* give repeated boluses.
  3. For PVCs in the presence of a bradycardia, give atropine 0.5 mg IV push.
- *For ventricular tachycardia* where the patient *is not perfusing:*
  1. Perform synchronized cardioversion at 200 w/s.
  2. After conversion to a supraventricular rhythm, give Lidocaine bolus and drip.
- *For ventricular fibrillation:*
  1. If arrest was unwitnessed, continue CPR for 2 minutes before attempting conversion.
  2. Defibrillate at 200–300 w/s (delivered); if no conversion, repeat immediately.
  3. If ineffective, give epinephrine 0.5–1 mg 1:10,000 IV push, via ET tube, or IC.
  4. Defibrillate a third time at a w/s setting not to exceed 360 joules (delivered).
  5. After conversion to a supraventricular rhythm, give Lidocaine bolus and drip.
- *For recurring* or *refractory ventricular fibrillation* which does not respond to other measures:

1. Give Bretylium 5 mg/kg rapid IV push; defibrillate; then give 10 mg/kg if needed.
2. Repeat if necessary at 15–30 minute intervals to a maximum of 30 mg/kg.
3. Follow with an IV drip of Bretylium 1–2 mg/minute.

Ventricular Bradyarrhythmias

- *For third degree heart blocks* at the ventricular level, or for *idioventricular rhythm:*
  1. Give atropine 0.5 mg IV push, *and/or,*
  2. Give Isuprel 2–20 mcg/minute.
- *For asystole* or *electromechanical dissociation:*
  1. Give Epinephrine 0.5–1 mg (1:10,000) IV push, via ET tube, or IC, *and/or*
  2. Give calcium chloride 5–7 mg/kg IV push; repeat every 10 minutes if necessary.
  3. If rhythm is not restored, administer up to 2 mg atropine IV push, and/or Isuprel 2–20 mcg/minute IV drip.

Special Note

- Cardiac arrhythmias are treated only if they are causing, or have the potential to cause, symptoms of decreased cardiac output.
- Treatments will not necessarily be initiated in this order, nor will all drugs/maneuvers listed be given for every arrhythmia, since arrhythmias with varying severity will require more or less aggressive treatments.
- All patients with arrhythmias (or the potential for them) should receive an IV of 5% D/W TKO. They will also require standard measures to ensure patency of airway, adequacy of ventilation, and especially oxygenation.
- All arrhythmias that cause cardiopulmonary arrest will require basic resuscitative measures, as well as sodium bicarbonate 1 mEq/kg IV push initially; thereafter, no more than one half the initial dose every 10–15 minutes for the remainder of the arrest. Effective CPR must be maintained. Antishock trousers can be used to enhance perfusion.
- Patients with myocardial infarction should not receive atropine for a bradycardia unless it is accompanied by decreased blood pressure or PVCs, or unless the rate falls below 50.

- A single precordial thump can be delivered immediately after recognizing ventricular tachycardia or ventricular fibrillation only if the patient was monitored and the arrhythmia noted immediately.

Pediatric Note

Pediatric doses:
- Valium: 0.25 mg/kg slow IV push over 3 minutes; may repeat once after 15–30 minutes; don't use in neonates less than 30 days old.
- Atropine: 0.01–0.03 mg/kg IV push, may repeat
- Isuprel: start at 0.1 mcg/kg/min IV drip
- Epinephrine: 0.01 ml/kg (1:10,000) IV push, via ET tube, IC
- Calcium chloride: 0.3 ml/kg (of 10% solution) IV push
- Lidocaine bolus: 1 mg/kg/dose; followed by drip of 30 mcg/kg/min
- Sodium bicarbonate: 1–2 mEq/kg/dose

Neither Digoxin, nor Bretylium should be given to children.

When defibrillating a child, use pediatric paddles or the anterior/posterior paddle placement; administer 2 w/s per kg initially; if unsuccessful, double this. If unsuccessful, give bicarbonate, epinephrine, and oxygen before increasing it further.

The precordial thump is not recommended in children.

Transport

- Monitor closely enroute.
- Watch drip rate on IV drugs; watch for side effects.
- No need for "red light and siren" if patient is stabilized.

ASTHMA

Asthma is a chronic lung disease characterized by bronchial constriction and an increase in thick mucuous production, resulting in impaired oxygen exchange. Acute attacks can be precipitated by allergic hypersensitivity to a foreign substance, or by psychological stress.

Signs and symptoms of acute asthma attack include dyspnea, restlessness, apprehension, prolonged expiratory phase, use of accessory muscles of respiration, wheezing, and tachycardia. This patient will usually be aware of his/her disease, and can give you pertinent historical information to guide treatment.

Treatment of acute attacks includes humidified high-flow oxygen and hydration to reduce viscosity and facilitate expulsion of mucuous plugs. A quiet environment is helpful, particularly if stress was a precipitator of the attack. In such a case, it might be helpful to remove the patient from family members or onlookers; consider moving the patient to the ambulance to begin treatment. In the presence of significant bronchial constriction, bronchodilators such as Isuprel Mistometer, Metaprel Inhalant, Epinephrine 1:1,000, and Aminophylline might be indicated. Most chronic asthma patients have a prescription for bronchodilator inhalants, so ask about prior use before administering additional drugs.

TREATMENT PROTOCOL: ASTHMA

History

- When did the respiratory difficulty start?
- Did it come on suddenly?
- What provoked the attack?
- How bad is this attack?
- Is the patient having trouble getting air in? Getting air out?
- Has this happened before?
- What usually breaks the attack?
- Has the patient taken any medications for this attack? If so, what? When?

Physical Exam

- What is the rate, depth, and quality of respiration?
- What is the level of consciousness?
- What is the skin color, temperature, and moisture?
- What are the patient's vital signs?
- What lung sounds are heart on auscultation?

- What is the EKG pattern?
- Are there any physical findings that might indicate an allergic reaction or congestive heart failure?

Differential Diagnosis

Rule out:
- allergic reaction
- upper airway obstruction
- congestive heart failure with pulmonary edema (cardiac asthma)

Can also be confused with:
- bronchitis/emphysema
- spontaneous pneumothorax
- pulmonary embolus
- hyperventilation syndrome

Treatment

1. Ensure airway and give high-flow humidified oxygen.
2. Allow patient to assume position of comfort.
3. Give Isuprel or Metaprel by inhalant.
4. Give Epinephrine 0.3 mg 1:1,000 SC; may repeat 3 times at 5-minute intervals.
5. Start an IV of 5% D/W TKO; may hydrate the patient with IV RL or NS, or oral fluids.
6. If Epinephrine is not effective, give Aminophylline 3–6 mg/kg in at least 20 ml 5% D/W IV Volutrol over a minimum of 20 minutes.

Special Note

- It is often helpful to move the patient into the ambulance and out of the public eye before treating; a quiet environment helps to calm the patient.
- If the patient took medication prior to arrival of the paramedics, bring the medication container.

Pediatric Note

- Pediatric dosage of Epinephrine 1:1,000 is 0.01 ml/kg SC; may repeat 3 times at 20 minute intervals to a maximum of 0.3 mg.
- Aminophylline should be used with caution in children.

Transport

- Transport patient in an upright position and give oxygen.
- If unable to relieve attack, transport the patient immediately in position of comfort.

BEHAVIORAL EMERGENCIES

A behavioral emergency exists when a patient demonstrates unusual, bizarre, or socially aberrant actions, ideas or moods which may result in disruption to himself or those around him. These conditions can be caused by mental or emotional problems, but can also be a manifestation of an organic medical disorder. In the emergency setting it is important to rule out the presence of an acute medical condition before assuming the patient has an emotional problem.

Acute medical disorders which can mimic behavioral emergencies include head injuries, diabetic imbalance, hypoxia and exposure to toxic substances. You might be able to eliminate some of these possibilities by giving oxygen or IV dextrose for differential diagnosis. However, in an emergency setting with an emotionally disturbed patient, it is often impractical to attempt such diagnostic maneuvers.

Behavior emergencies caused by acute alterations in mental or emotional balance usually fall into one of four categories:

Acute Psychiatric Disorders: Patients exhibiting severe emotional distress, depressive states, manic states, schizophrenia, paranoia, hysterical conversion reaction or catatonia.

Acute Alcohol Intoxication: Patients who have ingested quantities of alcohol beyond the body's tolerance level.

Acute Drug Intoxication: Patients who have ingested depressants, amphetamines, hallucinogens, or other thought-altering agents.

Withdrawal Syndrome: Patients in acute states of withdrawl from either alcohol or drugs.

Regardless of the cause of the behavioral disturbance, nearly all of these patients behave in one of two ways when encountered in the field:

Quiet: withdrawn, passive or suicidal

Aggressive: violent or combative

The primary responsibility of the paramedic is to transport the patient for appropriate medical care rather than performing extensive psychiatric interview in the field. Therefore, field management of these patients consists of getting the patient into the ambulance and to the hospital expediently, while preventing either physical or emotional harm to the patient. Approach to treatment is determined by whether the patient is quiet or aggressive.

The Quiet Patient

The quiet patient may be suffering from acute grief, schizophrenia, ingestion of barbiturates or other depressive drugs, depression, catatonia, hysterical conversion, manic states, or alcohol intoxication. Regardless of the cause, these patients respond best to a calm, direct manner, and active interest in their problem. An interested person who will provide support during this period of turmoil will often be able to stabilize the patient sufficiently to get him/her to the hospital.

The suicidal patient usually is included in this group but requires special consideration because his/her situation is so acute that death may be imminent. Convey to the patient that you are interested in his/her problem and that you sincerely want to help. Share your feelings and observations and try to convince the patient that you can help him/her deal with the situation. Avoid challenging commands, and don't underestimate or talk down to him/her. This type of patient is extremely perceptive; don't lie.

The Aggressive Patient

Aggressive patients present more of a challenge to the paramedic than those who are quiet, because any action could result in further chaos as well as possible injury to others at the scene. Several principles can be employed in managing violent patients. First realize that these patients are protecting themselves. Use of body language is important with this type of patient. Give them room. Don't make any moves that they may perceive as a threat. Don't stand between the patient and the door. Allow your body to assume a posture of relaxation, rather than confrontation. Don't stand directly in front of the patient; it is less threatening to sit or kneel off to one side. Allow the patient to vent feelings. Use his/her own words to describe the situation. If all else fails, it may be necessary to forcefully restrain the patient. Once this decision is made, don't discuss it openly, just move in with at least four people and restrain each extremity as rapidly as possible. Speak firmly but don't react to verbal abuse the patient may give you. Try to keep this action as calm as it can be. Keep the restraints on until you arrive at the hospital. Avoid a "red lights and siren" response since this will further stimulate the patient.

General Guidelines

Behavioral emergencies require paramedics to use their instincts in order to manage the patient. Although several principles are available to assist you, it will be your own gut feelings that guide you in these situations. Sometimes a hand placed gently on the shoulder will give the patient needed support and security; other times, the same gesture might be taken as a direct assault and will result in combative behavior. Keep in mind that your role is not to diagnose and solve the patient's problems; rather your primary goal is to get the patient safely and quickly to specialized medical care.

Several legal considerations are involved with behavioral emergencies. These include the validity of a consent form which is signed by an emotionally disturbed patient and the use of legal commitment to restrain and forcefully transport an unwilling patient. Learn the laws for your area and be aware of the resources available to you.

TREATMENT PROTOCOL: BEHAVIORAL EMERGENCIES

History

- What was the patient's behavior prior to your arrival?
- What was the patient doing at the time?
- What behavior is the patient exhibiting now?
- How long has this behavior been going on?
- Has this happened before?
- What is the mental status, including general appearance, affect, thought processes, and cognitive knowledge?
- Is there any indication of trauma?
- Has the patient taken any drugs or been drinking?

- Does the patient take any medications?
- Is there any history of mental illness?
- Is the patient seeing a personal physician?
- Is there any history of diabetes, hypertension, or seizure disorder?

Physical Exam

- Is there any respiratory distress?
- Is there any sign of head injury or other trauma?
- What is the level of consciousness?
- What are the vital signs?
- What is the skin temperature, color and moisture?
- What are the lung sounds?
- What are the pupils?
- What is the EKG pattern?
- Are there any needle marks?
- Is there a Medic-Alert tag or wallet card?

Differential Diagnosis

Rule out:
- hypoxia
- head injury
- drugs
- alcohol ingestion
- hypoglycemia
- CVA

Treatment

1. Ensure airway patency and give high-flow oxygen if possible.
2. Use a calm, firm approach with the patient.
3. Treat any associated injuries.
4. If hypoglycemia is suspected:
   a) Draw blood sugar.
   b) Give glucola, 75–100 Gm orally unless patient has a diminished gag reflex.

    c) Give 50% dextrose, 25 Gm IV push if unable to give oral glucose.

5. Consider Valium 2.5–20 mg IV push or IM for acute stress reaction.

6. If the patient is aggressive, use restraints as needed to protect the patient and others.

Special Note

- Patient is often a threat to himself or others. Approach will have to vary with each patient; it may not be practical to attempt history, physical or extensive treatment on these patients.
- The majority of patient management will come from individual interactions at the scene. It is very likely that communications will be interspersed with long pauses.
- Bring in any samples of ingested drugs, plants, or other causative agents.

Pediatric Note:

Pediatric dosages:
- Glucola: 10–100 Gm according to weight
- 50% Dextrose: 1 ml/kg slow IV push
- Valium: 0.25 mg/kg slow IV push over a 3-minute period; may repeat once after 15–30 minutes; don't use in neonates less than 30 days old

Transport:

- Restrain only if necessary to prevent injury.
- Avoid unnecessary "red lights and siren" response, as it can upset patient.
- Consider law enforcement assistance if needed.

BURNS

The skin regulates fluid loss, controls temperature, prevents infection, and contains sensory receptors. Burns destroy some or all layers of skin, thus interfering with these important functions. The severity and treatment of a burn are determined by the degree, extent, and source of the burn.

Degree of the Burn

A *first degree* burn is dry, painful, reddened, and blanches easily. It involves the epidermis only. A *second degree* burn has a moist surface, is red or mottled, has blisters, is painful, and blanches to pressure. It involves the epidermis and part of the dermis. *Third degree* burns are characterized as dry, hard and leathery, pearly white or charred, with congealed blood vessels and decreased pain secondary to destruction of nerve endings.

It is often quite difficult to determine the degree of the burn initially, but you should attempt to estimate it as accurately as possible. Regardless of the source of a burn, the degree is determined by the foregoing criteria.

Extent of the Burn

The extent of a burn, i.e., the size of the area affected, is calculated in an adult by using the "Rule of Nines." Due to different body proportions a modified chart is used for children.

Both methods of estimating burned surface area are illustrated in Figure 1.1

Source of the Burn

A *thermal burn* is any burn caused by heat, e.g., flame, steam, or liquid. When such burns occur skin layers, blood vessels, and nerve endings may be destroyed. In addition, the capillaries in the burned area weaken and lose their permeability, allowing fluid and plasma proteins to escape from the circulatory system into the interstitial and extracellular spaces (the "third space"). If this displaced circulatory volume is not restored, hypovolemic shock will result.

Field management of thermal burns begins with the assurance that you and your patient are out of danger. Make sure the fire is extinguished and the clothing is not smoldering. Follow the ABCs with high-flow oxygen, determine whether or not there is respiratory involvement, and assess any associated injuries. Depending on the extent and degree of burn, volume IV fluid replacement with RL or NS may be indicated.

Pain may be present in minor first and second degree burns. If so, saline soaks or ice packs may be beneficial in reducing pain. However, the ice

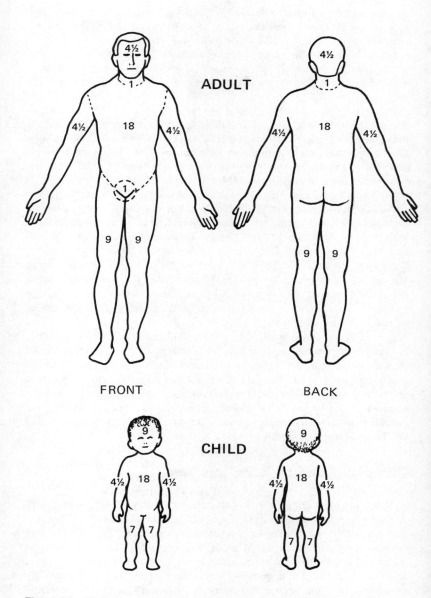

Figure 1.1. Illustrates the "Rule of Nines" used to estimate body surface area involvement of burn injuries in an adult and the modification for children under five.

should not be in direct contact with the skin. Morphine sulfate in small increments IV may be necessary for relief of pain if the patient doesn't respond to reassurance and other basic measures.

Dress the wounds in sterile or clean bandages. While wet dressings may be appropriate for small burns, they can contribute to hypothermia in major burns. For this reason use dry dressings for burns of large surface area.

Frequent evaluation of vital signs and respiratory status is important, as is a good history and physical examination. Remove all rings, watches, necklaces, and other constrictive articles. Don't give any fluids orally. Don't apply any grease or ointment to the burns, don't break any blisters, and don't remove any clothing that is stuck to burned tissue. Do not administer any medications by IM route.

Chemical burns cause a pathological state similar to thermal burns, but are usually more localized. Basically, these burns are treated the same as a thermal injury, except that the chemical must first be removed by flushing with copious amounts of water. Use extreme care to avoid personal contact with the chemical. Because the chemical can continue burning for some time, the area must be flushed continuously during transport. If large body areas are involved, the patient should be placed in a shower or hosed off. If the chemical is a dry powder, brush off as much as possible before hosing the patient with water. Remove clothing carefully to prevent further exposure to the chemical.

Electrical burns are unique because, in addition to surface burns, there is a danger of internal damage along the pathways of the electrical current. Respiratory arrest or ventricular fibrillation can occur secondary to the electrical current itself. Field treatment follows the same principles as that of thermal burns, but with emphasis on respiratory and cardiovascular support. Always start an IV and monitor EKG as a precautionary measure. Electrical burns are very serious and should always be transported to the hospital for evaluation.

Complications of Burn Injuries

Many burn patients have associated *respiratory involvement* which further complicates their injury. Early recognition of pulmonary burns is essential. Pulmonary involvement should be suspected if the burn occurs within an enclosed area, involves the face or neck, or results in singed facial and nasal hairs or soot or blisters in the nose, mouth, or oropharynx. Initially, a patient with respiratory involvement may have normal respirations, but as burn edema and bronchial irritation increase, signs and symptoms of dyspnea, hoarseness, cough, and cyanosis may be seen. Do not use MS if pulmonary involvement is suspected and be prepared to intubate if laryngeal edema is anticipated. Give high-flow humidified oxygen and transport promptly.

Carbon monoxide (CO) poisoning should be suspected in all patients found unconscious at the scene of a fire, or any patient burned in an enclosed area. Signs and symptoms include headache, weakness, tingling in the extremities, confusion, reckless behavior, collapse and coma. Cyanosis can be masked because of the effect carbon monoxide has on the mucous membranes. The cherry-red coloring often attributed to CO poisoning is a late characteristic, and thus is an unreliable early field sign. Treatment for CO poisoning is to remove the patient from the source of the gas and then hyperventilate with high-flow oxygen to help blow off the carbon monoxide.

While *infection* is a leading cause of death following a major burn, it generally does not appear for 24–48 hours. In the field, you can help prevent this complication by keeping the burned area as clean as possible. Another complication is *corneal abrasion,* which frequently occurs following flash burns of the face. Signs and symptoms include a scratchy feeling, blurred vision, or clouding of the cornea. Treatment consists of saline irrigation and patching.

Determining Need for Transport

You will frequently be in a position to witness patients with very minor burns which do not need to be rushed to a hospital, but instead can be seen by a private physician. However, some burns can appear minor but still need immediate specialized care to prevent long-term disability or even death. As a general rule, patients requiring transport are those with:

- Second and third degree burns over 15–30% of the body
- Involvement of critical areas (hands, face, feet, genitalia)
- Respiratory involvement
- Associated soft tissue injury and/or fractures
- Electrical injuries
- Very young or very old patients

TREATMENT PROTOCOL: BURNS

History

- What was the causative agent (heat, chemical, electricity)?
- Where, when and how did the burn occur?

- Was the patient burned in an enclosed space such as a car or garage?
- What is the patient's age and weight?
- What is the patient's medical history?
- Was any treatment instituted prior to your arrival?

Physical Exam

- Are there any signs of respiratory distress?
- Are there any signs of laryngeal edema?
- Is there any sign suggestive of respiratory involvement such as singed nasal hairs, burns of the face, or soot or blisters in the oropharynx?
- What is the patient's level of consciousness?
- What are the vital signs?
- What are the lung sounds on auscultation?
- Where are the burns located?
- What is the estimated percentage and degree of the burn injury?
- Are there any associated injuries?
- If electrical, is there an entrance or exit wound?
- If chemical, what agent was involved?

Differential Diagnosis

- Rule out respiratory involvement
- Rule out carbon monoxide poisoning
- Determine severity of burn:

  Major: over 20% second or third degree; or respiratory involvement; or underlying disease (heart, respiratory)

  Minor: less than 20% second or third degree; and no respiratory involvement or complicating factors

Treatment

1. Move patient to a safe environment
2. Break contact with causative agent (extinguish flames, wash off chemicals).

3. Ensure airway, give oxygen, and ventilate if necessary.
4. Treat associated injuries.
5. If burn is *Major:*
   a. Start an IV or RL or NS and run to maintain blood pressure.
   b. If necessary, give morphine sulfate 2–5 mg IV push, may repeat every 5–30 minutes.
   c. Cover wounds.
   d. Keep patient warm.
6. If burn is *Minor:*
   a. Apply cool saline soaks to help alleviate pain.
   b. Cover wound.
   c. Keep patient warm.
   d. May start an IV of RL or NS TKO as a precaution.
7. Do not break blisters, remove stuck clothing, soak wounded area in ice water, apply any type of ointment, or give any IM medications.
8. Remove all constricting items such as rings, necklaces, and bracelets.

For Chemical Burns: Flush immediately with copious amounts of water. If the chemical is dry, brush it off before flushing. Use caution to prevent personal exposure.

For Electrical Burns: Treat symptomatically. Support cardiovascular system and monitor closely.

For Respiratory Burns: Intubate if necessary; transport immediately.

For Tar Burns: Cool with water and transport. Do not attempt to remove the tar.

Special Note

- If the patient is unconscious, consider head injury or carbon monoxide poisoning.

Pediatric Note

- Pediatric dosage of morphine: 0.1–0.2 mg/kg IV push over 3–5 minutes; titrate to effect.
- Body surface area is estimated differently in children than adults.
- Burns are one of the more common forms of child abuse.

Transport

- Transport immediately to nearest basic emergency facility if the patient has respiratory involvement.
- Follow triage guidelines to determine most appropriate facility for care.
- Any burn of a critical area such as hands, feet, face or perineum should be transported for medical evaluation regardless of how small the affected area.

CARDIAC ARREST

Cardiopulmonary arrest is defined as cessation of both cardiac and respiratory function. Respiratory arrest can occur alone as a result of drug overdose, airway obstruction, suffocation, electrocution, trauma, neurological disorder, or near-drowning. Cardiac arrest with concurrent respiratory arrest can take the form of ventricular fibrillation, ventricular tachycardia, asystole, or cardiovascular collapse (electromechanical dissociation.)

Confirming Cardiac Arrest

The initial assessment step is to determine adequacy of airway, breathing, and circulation. Findings consistent with full cardiac arrest include loss of consciousness and absence of respirations, pulses, and blood pressure. Cyanosis and dilated pupils follow quickly. Skeletal muscle seizures, vomiting, and urinary/fecal incontinence are common. Steps in confirming cardiopulmonary arrest are:

1. Establish unresponsiveness (shake and shout).
2. Open airway, establish breathlessness (look, listen, feel).
3. Establish absence of pulse.

Cardiopulmonary Resuscitation (CPR)

The cardiac arrest patient is initially managed with cardiopulmonary resuscitation. CPR should not be initiated if the patient is known to have been in arrest for longer than ten minutes, is suffering from an incurable disease in terminal stages, or is obviously dead from major trauma such as decapitation. When uncertain whether or not to initiate CPR, give the patient the benefit of the doubt and start CPR.

Any deficiencies in vital body functions noted in the initial assessment must be corrected immediately before proceeding with more sophisticated assessment or intervention. The critical steps in gaining control of vital functions are:

Airway: Open and clear airway, using spinal precautions if indicated. As soon as possible, insert an esophageal obturator airway or endotracheal tube.

Breathing: Begin artificial ventilation, using mouth-to-mouth breathing or an Ambu bag initially, and switching to a demand valve as soon as possible. Supplement with 100% oxygen.

Circulation: Begin external cardiac compression. Be certain patient is positioned on a hard, flat surface.

As soon as possible, obtain assistance from other personnel. Assess effectiveness of CPR by monitoring peripheral pulses and adequacy of ventilations. Meanwhile, attempt to get a pertinent medical history that may provide clues to the cause of the arrest; look for a correctable cause such as drug overdose or airway obstruction.

Intervention

Once the ABCs are controlled, you can begin corrective measures. Specific therapy will be guided by the cause of the arrest, if known. General management principles are outlined below:

1. *Monitor EKG:* Use the defibrillator's "quick-look" capability to identify cardiac rhythm; defibrillate if ventricular fibrillation. Attach monitoring electrodes and maintain close surveillance of rhythm changes. Position monitor for optimum visibility.

2. *Start an IV:* Use 5% D/W and run at a TKO rate. Select a large, stable vein if possible, and secure it well in anticipation of defibrillation.

3. *Correct Acidosis:* Respiratory acidosis can be controlled by adequate ventilation, but if the patient was in respiratory arrest, metabolic acidosis probably exists also. To correct metabolic acidosis, give sodium bicarbonate at prescribed intervals throughout the arrest.

4. *Treat Arrhythmias:* Treat presenting arrhythmias according to the Arrhythmia Protocol. Since most patients encounter many rhythm changes during the course of an arrest, it is best to use drug therapy conservatively to avoid overloading the patient.

5. *Support Perfusion:* Position patient with legs elevated to facilitate venous return. Antishock trousers can be applied for the

same effect. Dopamine is the drug of choice to maintain blood pressure, but vasopressors might be used instead.

Cardiac Arrest Following Trauma

Trauma-induced cardiac arrest presents special management problems. Special care must be taken to protect the spinal cord, especially when opening the airway and ventilating. A modified jaw thrust maneuver is used to keep the head and neck immobile while opening the airway. The entire spine should be immobilized as soon as possible to prevent movement during the resuscitation process. In addition to attending to the standard resuscitative procedures, the trauma patient requires control of bleeding and IV fluid volume replacement. Prompt transport is critical in trauma-induced cardiac arrest. Resuscitation efforts center around surgical intervention, and chances for survival are slim unless the patient receives immediate surgical attention.

Terminating Resuscitative Efforts

Cardiopulmonary resuscitation should only be terminated if:

a. the patient regains spontaneous respirations and pulses, or
b. the rescuer is relieved by someone of equal or higher medical qualifications, or
c. the rescuer is exhausted and cannot continue.

Once advanced resuscitative measures have been instituted, it is best to continue your efforts until you arrive at the hospital and are relieved by the emergency physician.

TREATMENT PROTOCOL: CARDIAC ARREST

History

- What happened?
- Was trauma involved?
- How long has the patient been down?
- What is the patient's age and weight?
- Does the patient have any terminal illness?
- Does the patient have a history of heart problems or other medical illness?

- Is the patient on any medications?
- What was the patient doing at the time of the attack?
- Was any treatment instituted prior to arrival of the paramedics?

Physical Exam

- What is the patient's level of consciousness?
- Is the patient breathing?
- What is the carotid pulse?
- What is the skin color, temperature, and moisture?
- What rhythm does the EKG paddle-check show?
- Are there any obvious injuries?

Differential Diagnosis

- Evaluate respirations and major pulses to determine if the patient has actually arrested.
- Determine whether the arrest was trauma-induced.

Treatment

1. Open airway; insert EOA or ET tube.
2. Ventilate with 100% oxygen by demand valve.
3. Begin cardiac compressions.
4. Control major bleeding.
5. Start an IV of 5% D/W TKO; if hypovolemia is suspected, use RL or NS and run to maintain blood pressure.
6. Administer sodium bicarbonate 1 mEq/kg initially; thereafter, give no more than one half that dose every 10–15 minutes of continued arrest.
7. Treat arrhythmias according to Arrhythmia Protocol.
8. Elevate legs or apply antishock trousers; to maintain blood pressure, give:
   - Dopamine 200 mg in 500 ml 5% D/W (400 mcg/ml) IV drip; begin with 2–5 mcg/kg/min, *or*
   - Aramine 100 mg in 250 ml 5% D/W; start at 0.4 mg/min, *or*
   - Levophed 8 mg in 500 ml 5% D/W (16 mcg/ml) IV drip; start at 2–3 ml/min. Titrate to blood pressure.
9. Treat underlying cause of arrest, if known.

Special Note

- Assess peripheral pulses, respiratory effectiveness, and pupils throughout resuscitation.
- Cardiac arrest following trauma is usually accompanied by hypovolemia and should be treated concurrently with antishock procedures.

Pediatric Note

Pediatric dosages:
- sodium bicarbonate: 1–2 mEq/kg IV push
- dopamine: 2–10 mcg/kg/min
- Aramine: 50–100 mg in 250 ml 5% D/W; start at 0.4 mg/kg
- Levophed: start at 0.1 mcg/kg/min

Children remain viable longer than adults, so may institute CPR even if the child has been down longer than 4–6 minutes.

Precordial thump is not recommended for children.

Transport

- Transport "red lights and sirens" as soon as possible.

CEREBROVASCULAR ACCIDENT

Cerebrovascular accident (CVA), also referred to as stroke, is a result of a thrombus, embolus, or hemorrhage which occludes the blood supply to a portion of the brain causing ischemia and/or infarction. Contributing factors include hypertension, atherosclerosis, thrombi, emboli, aneurysms, intracranial masses, and the use of birth control pills or anticoagulants. The patient's history may also include chronic atrial fibrillation or myocardial infarction.

CVAs are usually of sudden onset and may have been preceded by a headache. In the immediate post–injury stage, the blood pressure usually remains high, but may possibly be in the normal or low range. Signs and symptoms are related to the area of the brain where the damage has occurred. These may include unilateral paralysis and/or muscle weakness, aphasia, drooping of the mouth, drooling, incontinence, and occasionally unconsciousness or unequal pupils. The patient may have central respiratory involvement but this rarely occurs.

A disorder similar to CVA is *transient ischemic attack* (TIA). This condition is caused by cerebral vascular spasms or microemboli which produce many of the same symptoms as a CVA. TIA differs from CVA only in that its effects are temporary. The patient with TIA may be fully recovered by the time medical help arrives. Even though the patient may appear asymptomatic, all suspected TIAs should be transported for further medical evaluation, as it may be indicative of impending CVA.

Management of CVA and TIA

There is no relevant difference in management of symptomatic TIA and CVA patients in the prehospital setting. Airway control may require the insertion of an oral or nasopharyngeal airway and suction should be readily available. Position the patient on the side to reduce chances of aspiration if he/she has an altered level of consciousness, uncontrollable drooling or a decreased gag reflex from paralysis. Administer oxygen to combat any associated hypoxia and monitor the EKG for possible arrhythmias. Start an IV at a TKO rate in case medications are needed. D50W may be given diagnostically to rule out hypoglycemia, which can mimic the signs and symptoms associated with a CVA. Reassess vital signs, neurological status, and level of consciousness frequently during transport. Don't overlook the possibility of other associated injuries.

TREATMENT PROTOCOL: CEREBROVASCULAR ACCIDENT

History

- What is the problem?
- When did the problem start?
- What was the patient doing when the symptoms occurred?
- Did the patient have any headache, dizziness, or chest pain prior to the episode?
- Does the patient have any predisposing factors such as hypertension, atherosclerosis, prior CVAs or TIAs, recent illnesses or surgeries?

- Has the patient been taking any medication (especially anti-hypertensive agents, anticoagulants, or birth control pills)?
- Did the patient lose consciousness; if so, for how long?
- Has there been any change in level of consciousness since the symptoms began?
- Did the patient fall?
- Does the patient have a history of atrial fibrillation?
- Was there any seizure activity?

Physical Exam

- What is the respiratory rate, rhythm and effectiveness?
- What is the patient's level of consciousness?
- What is the patient's neorological status (pupils, hand grasps, movement of extremities, sensation)?
- Is there any facial paralysis, difficulty speaking, swallowing, or drooling?
- Has the patient been incontinent of urine or stool?
- What are the vital signs, lung sounds, skin color, temperature, and moisture?
- What is the EKG pattern?
- Is there any evidence of trauma?

Differential Diagnosis

- Hypoglycemia
- Seizure Disorder
- If the patient is unconscious, rule out other causes of coma.

Treatment

1. Ensure airway patency, given oxygen and ventilate if necessary.
2. If associated trauma, splint as necessary.
3. If patient is having difficulty with secretions, position on affected side and suction secretions.
4. Draw blood sugar.

5. Start IV TKO.
6. Administer 25 gm 50% dextrose IV push.
7. Reassure patient, especially if experiencing aphasia.

Transport

- Protect airway and watch for changes in patient status.

CHEST PAIN
(NON-TRAUMATIC)

Two types of clinical disorders cause pain in the region of the chest. These two categories are cardiovascular disorders and pulmonary disorders.

Cardiovascular Pain

The most common cardiovascular emergencies which present with chest pain are angina pectoris, myocardial infarction, aortic aneurysm, and pericarditis.

Angina Pectoris presents pain as a reflection of myocardial hypoxia, usually the result of increased oxygen demand and increased cardiac output. It can also be caused by arterial spasm or partial coronary artery occlusion. Angina produces chest pain very similar to that of myocardial infarction. The pain involves the substernal chest area, but may radiate to the arms, neck, or jaw. It is usually described as crushing, heavy, aching, or burning. The pain usually is aggravated by exercise, and can last from 1–5 minutes. In severe forms of angina, the pain can be more severe, last longer, and cause the patient to be diaphoretic and weak. The EKG shows transient ST depression which goes away with relief of pain. The objectives of treatment are to increase coronary blood flow and/or reduce oxygen demand. In addition to rest and oxygen, nitroglycerine is usually effective in controlling anginal pain.

Myocardial Infarction (MI) is defined as the death of a portion of heart muscle, most often due to occlusion of a coronary artery by plaque build-up or a thrombus. The usual presentation includes severe substernal chest pain which is a clinical manifestation of myocardial anoxia. The patient may deny actual pain, but will refer to it instead as pressure, indigestion, or a crushing sensation that came on suddenly, and which may have radiated down one or both arms, or up into the jaw or neck. Other signs and symptoms include cool clammy skin, diaphoresis, and nausea or vomiting. Depending on the severity of the damage, the patient may also have evidence of CHF and/or cardiogenic shock due to decreased effectiveness of the left ventricle.

The patient with an MI is subject to a wide range of arrhythmias which may be the result of either direct injury to the conduction system or underlying myocardial hypoxia. These arrhythmias can range from sinus bradycardia to ventricular fibrillation, and are the leading cause of death in this type of patient. Because the MI patient has such potential for lethal arrhythmias it is imperative that you immediately attach a cardiac monitor and promptly treat any arrhythmias that have the potential to cause a drop in cardiac output. Premature ventricular contractions and ventricular tachycardia are commonly seen in association with MIs and should be treated with lidocaine immediately. You should also consider the pro-phylactic use of lidocaine in the field management of all MI patients to prevent primary ventricular fibrillation. Watch for bradycardias and heart blocks, as the SA and AV nodes may be temporarily damaged. If atropine is required, it should be used cautiously, as an excessive rate increase can extend the infarct.

Any patient with chest pain should be treated as an MI until proven otherwise. Administer oxygen at a high flow-rate to increase oxygen supply to the heart, but be cautious with patients who have chronic lung disease. Start an IV of 5% D/W TKO for possible administration of medications. Morphine sulfate can be given in small increments to help relieve the pain and reduce the patient's anxiety. It is important to calm the patient as soon as possible to prevent any undue workload on the heart. Take vital signs as needed with particular emphasis on heart rate and blood pressure. Frequent reassessment of lung sounds is also essential because the patient with a large MI can progress very rapidly to CHF and pulmonary edema.

The MI patient can develop *cardiogenic shock*, an impairment of the heart muscle as a pump, which causes decreased tissue perfusion. It most often follows a massive MI, but can also be caused by sustained tachycar-dia, acute valvular insufficiency, pericardial tamponade, pulmonary em-bolus, tension pneumothorax, or end-stage CHF with pulmonary edema. Signs and symptoms include restlessness, anxiety, mental sluggishness, cool clammy skin, pallor, tachycardia, rapid shallow respirations, thirst, and severe hypotension. Treatment is aimed at improving tissue oxygena-tion and increasing the efficiency of the heart as a pump. Field treatment of cardiogenic shock includes high-flow oxygen, an IV of 5% D/W TKO, dopamine or vasopressors, arrhythmia suppression as needed, and treat-ment of associated injuries or illnesses. This is a critical condition and warrants very close monitoring of vital signs and EKG.

When preparing for transport, don't allow the MI patient to walk to the guerney. Keep oxygen on enroute, and avoid a "red lights and siren" response. Continue to reassure the patient, because this condition is often accompanied by a feeling of impending death.

Aortic Aneurysm is caused by a tear in the inner lining of the aorta that allows blood to leak in between the vessel layers. Extension of the separation of linings (dissection) can cause occlusion of the major vessels that branch off the aorta. This condition is usually associated with hypertension, arteriosclerotic heart disease, or trauma. The predominant symptom of dissecting aneurysm is its characteristic pain. Located in the anteroposterior chest area, it is often described as excruciating, knife-like, or tearing. The patient will be extremely anxious, and can experience dyspnea, diaphoresis, pallor, tachycardia, and syncope. If the aneurysm ruptures into the pericardial sac it can cause cardiac tamponade. More likely, it will rupture into the chest cavity and cause rapid exsanguination. Treatment includes aggressive antishock measures and prompt transport; surgical intervention is required, although mortality rate is very high.

Pericarditis is defined as an inflammation of the pericardial sac. It is most often caused by infection, trauma, or coronary artery disease. It is characterized by chest pain associated with respiration or increased activity. Other signs and symptoms include fever and chills, dyspnea, tachycardia, diaphoresis, malaise, and possibly hypotension. The ST segment on the EKG can be elevated, and chest auscultation might reveal a pericardial friction rub. Field treatment is limited, including oxygen and possibly analgesia or sedation. Hospitalization is required to provide rest and antibiotic therapy.

Respiratory Pain

The most common respiratory emergencies which present with chest pain are pulmonary embolism, spontaneous pneumothorax, pleurisy, and pneumonia.

Pulmonary embolism occurs when a blood clot travels from one part of the body and lodges in a pulmonary vessel, occluding circulation to a portion of the lungs. Predisposing factors to pulmonary embolism include inactivity, recent surgery, pregnancy, varicose veins, or use of birth control pills. Signs and symptoms are dependent on the amount of tissue damage, but can include pleuritic chest pain of sudden onset, dyspnea, diaphoresis, hemoptysis, fever, cyanosis, and profound shock in severe cases. Treatment consists of high-flow oxygen, an IV of 5% D/W TKO, symptomatic life support, and prompt transport.

Spontaneous pneumothorax is a partially or totally collapsed lung, the result of a ruptured bleb on the pleural lining. It occurs without warning and most commonly strikes young adult males. It can frequently be identified by sudden onset of dyspnea, cough, and a sharp chest pain which might be referred to the shoulder. Breath sounds can be diminished or absent on the affected side. Field treatment is supportive, and may include ventilatory assistance, an IV of 5% D/W TKO, and monitoring of EKG.

Pleurisy is an inflammation of the lining of the lung causing localized pain on inspiration due to the pleura rubbing against each other. Respirations are usually rapid and shallow as the patient attempts to splint breathing and reduce the pain. Once again, treatment consists of high-flow oxygen, an IV of 5% D/W TKO, and supportive care.

Pneumonia is an inflammatory process involving the alveoli. It can be caused by bacteria, virus, or aspiration. Signs and symptoms include fever, cough with large amounts of dark-colored sputum, chest pain on inspiration, flushed face, weak and rapid pulse, and dyspnea. In advanced cases, rales, rhonchi, and areas of decreased breath sounds can be heard on auscultation. Field treatment is limited, but might include oxygen, an IV of 5% D/W TKO, close monitoring, and symptomatic support.

TREATMENT PROTOCOL: CHEST PAIN (NON-TRAUMATIC)

History

- When did the chest pain start?
- How does the patient describe the pain?
- How severe is the pain?
- Where is the pain located, and does it radiate to arms, back, neck, jaw, or shoulder?
- What was the patient doing when the pain started?
- Is the pain associated with respiration or difficulty breathing?
- Does anything make the pain better or worse?
- Has this ever happened before?
- What is the patient's medical history?
- Is the patient taking any medication?
- Has the patient taken anything for the chest pain?
- Is the patient nauseated?

Physical Exam

- Is the patient breathing effectively?
- What is the level of consciousness?

- What is the skin color, moisture, and temperature?
- What are the vital signs?
- Are blood pressures and pulses equal bilaterally?
- What is the EKG pattern?
- What are the lung sounds?
- Is the pain associated with respiration or movement of the chest wall?
- Are there any signs of CHF such as distended neck veins or peripheral edema?

Differential Diagnosis

- Rule out trauma.

Treatment

1. Ensure airway; assist respirations if necessary.
2. Give high-flow oxygen.
3. Start an IV of 5% D/W TKO. If hypovolemia is suspected (as with ruptured aneurysm) use RL or NS and run to maintain blood pressure.
4. Monitor EKG; treat arrhythmias according to Arrhythmia Protocol.
5. Transport promptly, providing symptomatic life support as appropriate.

For Angina Pectoria

a. Give nitroglycerine 0.4 mg (1/150 gr) sublingually; may repeat at 3–5 minute intervals as necessary, up to a total of 3 tablets.
b. If no relief, give morphine in 2–5 mg increments slow IV push; may repeat every 5–30 minutes, titrate to effect.

For Myocardial Infarction

a. Give morphine sulfate in 2–5 mg increments IV push to relief of pain.
b. Give prophylatic lidocaine, 200 mg initial loading dose, IV push; follow with repeated boluses or IV drip.
c. If patient is hypotensive and cardiogenic shock is suspected, give:

- dopamine 200 mg in 500 ml 5% D/W (400 mcg/ml) IV drip; start with 2–5 mcg/kg/min, *or*
- aramine 100 mg in 250 ml 5% D/W IV drip; start with 0.4 mg/min, *or*
- levophed 8 mg in 500 ml 5% D/W IV drip (16 mcg/ml), start at 2–3 ml/min.

Titrate to blood pressure.

For Aneurysm

a. Start IV with RL or NS using large bore cannula needle. Run to maintain blood pressure.
b. Transport immediately, instituting aggressive antishock measures enroute.

For Pericarditis

a. Consider analgesics or sedatives for pain.
b. Transport for antibiotic therapy.

Special Note

- Patients who complain of chest pain in the field should be suspected of having had an MI and be treated accordingly unless evidence negates this possibility.
- Cardiogenic shock carries a high mortality rate and warrants immediate attention.

Transport

- Do not use "red lights and siren" unless condition is critical.
- Allow patient to assume position of comfort during transport.

CHEST TRAUMA

Any trauma severe enough to threaten the integrity of the thoracic cage is likely to cause concurrent damage to the underlying structures as well. Even if the chest wall remains intact, there is still a strong possibility of injury to the heart, lungs, and/or major blood vessels. When the injury is to the lower thorax, it can also involve organs of the upper abdominal cavity.

Cardiac Trauma

Frequently, the only early warning of cardiac trauma is a suspicious mechanism of injury such as chest impact with a steering wheel. Other signs which may substantiate your suspicions include rib fractures or bruising over the pericardium. Some of the more common types of cardiac trauma are discussed in the following paragraphs.

Cardiac Contusion results from direct blunt trauma to the heart, and can present as cardiac insufficiency or as a myocardial infarction. The patient may complain of chest pain, and the EKG can reveal ST changes or arrhythmias. Treatment includes high-flow oxygen and support of vital functions. Due to possible ventricular damage, arrhythmias are likely and should be treated as necessary with antiarrhythmic agents. Don't overlook the possibility of an underlying MI as a possible cause of the original trauma.

Pericardial Tamponade occurs when blood accumulates in the pericardial space and suppresses the pumping action of the heart. This condition can result from either blunt or penetrating trauma to the chest wall. Signs and symptoms include tachycardia, hypotension, distension of neck veins, cyanosis, muffled heart sounds, and profound shock. Immediate pericardiocentesis to remove accumulated blood from the pericardial sac is the treatment of choice. If you are medically or legally unauthorized to perform this procedure in the field, transport immediately and support vital functions enroute.

Ventricular Rupture can cause rapid exsanguination and profound circulatory collapse. This situation requires immediate transport, with massive volume restoration and antishock trousers enroute. Chances for survival are very slim.

Pulmonary Trauma

Trauma to the chest wall frequently disrupts the structural integrity of the respiratory system, thereby interfering with normal air exchange. The resulting hypoxia can produce cerebral symptoms (i.e., seizures, coma) or cardiovascular manifestations (i.e., arrhythmias, arrest). The more common types of pulmonary trauma are discussed below.

Traumatic Pneumothorax/Hemothorax occurs when either air or blood enters the pleural cavity following trauma, resulting in a partial or complete collapse of one or both lungs. These disorders are commonly caused by fractured ribs, and usually render the patient dyspneic. Other signs include bruising of the chest wall and crepitus in the affected area. Often associated with the severe dyspnea is pain on inspiration and guarded respirations. Upon auscultation, breath sounds may be diminished on the affected side or increased on the opposite side depending on the extent of lung involvement. Subcutaneous emphysema may also be present. Field treatment is directed toward supporting respirations and preventing shock. Give high-flow oxygen, monitor EKG, check for associated injuries and immobilize as needed. Start an IV for possible fluid volume replacement. Assist ventilations as necessary and watch closely for possible progression to tension pneumothorax.

Tension Pneumothorax is created by an opening in the chest wall with a one-way flap that allows air to enter the pleural cavity but does not allow air to escape. This alters intrathoracic pressure and creates an internal tension which increases with each breath. This condition should be suspected when a patient becomes increasingly dyspneic and anxious with each respiration. As the condition progresses, more air fills the affected side, and the trachea may shift to the opposite side along with the mediastinum. If allowed to continue, the pressure can compress the good lung and hinder respirations. This tension causes the heart and great vessels to be shifted and compressed, thus altering circulatory status by preventing blood from returning to the heart. The classic presentation includes restlessness and anxiety, increasing dyspnea, tracheal and/or mediastinal shifting, cyanosis, and distended neck veins.

Although tension pneumothorax can be fatal if left untreated, it rarely progresses to a life-threatening stage in less time than it takes to transport the patient. Therefore, it may be more appropriate to transport the patient than to initiate invasive field treatment unless the transport time is unusually long. If the patient is suffering from tension pneumothorax and requires immediate relief, a needle thoracostomy may be indicated. Assist respirations as needed, give high-flow oxygen, and start an IV TKO. Since this patient frequently has associated trauma, use RL or NS, and increase flow rate if hypovolemia is suspected. Monitor vital signs and EKG, and transport promptly.

Flail Chest exists when two or more contiguous ribs are each fractured in two places, thus creating a floating section and preventing the chest wall from expanding adequately for ventilation. Paradoxical respirations will be present resulting in impaired respiratory function. The patient will exhibit extreme anxiety with dyspnea, tachycardia, and possibly cyanosis. Treatment is aimed at stabilizing the chest wall with support to the injured side in order to facilitate ventilation. This can best be done by placing the victim on the injured side and/or splinting the affected side with sandbags. Following this, the patient should be ventilated with a positive-pressure resuscitator and intubated if necessary. Check for associated injuries, immobilize the spine, monitor cardiac and respiratory status, and start an IV or RL or NS. Volume replacement may be necessary if hypovolemia is present. Watch closely for evidence of progression to tension pneumothorax and transport promptly.

Open Chest Injuries refers to penetrating injury to the chest wall, wherein air is allowed to enter the pleural cavity, causing extreme respiratory distress, cyanosis, and a sucking sound with each inspiration. A common treatment for this "sucking chest wound" is to seal it with a Vasoline gauze dressing. However, this might convert the injury to a tension pneumothorax. If the patient becomes increasingly dyspneic following application of the dressing, remove it to allow release of internal pressure; then reseal the wound. Support respiratory and cardiovascular status as necessary and transport quickly. If a penetrating object is protruding from the wound, leave it in place and stabilize it with bandages. However, should CPR be necessary, the protruding object should be removed to prevent further damage.

Vascular Trauma

Trauma to the great vessels is usually caused by rapid acceleration/ deceleration accidents. In severe cases, the blood vessels are torn completely from the myocardium. Immediate, profound exsanguination occurs, mandating rapid transport with aggressive antishock measures enroute. When the trauma is less devastating, the patient may respond to standard antishock measures, including oxygen, IV volume replacement, and antishock trousers. Even minimal injury such as a small tear or separation presents a major threat to life, and prompt transport is critical.

TREATMENT PROTOCOL: CHEST TRAUMA

History

- What was the mechanism of injury?
- What is the nature and extent of injuries?
- Is the patient having any respiratory distress?
- Is there any pain; if so, where?
- Is there any cough or hemoptysis?
- Does the patient have any major medical illness?

Physical Exam

- Is the airway adequate?
- Are respirations effective?

- Is there any bleeding?
- Is there any paradoxical respiration, intercostal indrawing, tracheal deviation, or neck vein distention?
- What is the skin color, temperature, and moisture?
- What are the vital signs?
- What is the level of consciousness?
- What are the lung sounds?
- What is the EKG pattern?
- What are the findings of a head-to-toe exam?

Differential Diagnosis

- Differentiate between cardiac, pulmonary, and vascular trauma.
- Rule out involvement of upper abdominal organs.

Treatment

1. Ensure patent airway; intubate if needed; use suction and positioning to keep airway open; keep spine immobile if at all possible.
2. Give high-flow oxygen; ventilate if necessary.
3. Correct any structural defects in respiratory system; cover open chest wounds, stabilize floating rib sections, etc.
5. Control any active bleeding.
6. Start an IV of RL or NS TKO. Increase rate if hypovolemia is suspected. If shock is present, implement standard antishock measures.
7. Do not administer analgesics.
8. Treat associated injuries; transport promptly.

For Cardiac Tamponade: Perform a pericardiocentesis if authorized, or transport immediately "red lights and siren."

For Tension Pneumothorax: Perform a needle thoracostomy if authorized, or transport immediately "red lights and siren."

For Open Chest Wound: Cover with Vasoline gauze but watch for development of tension pneumothorax; remove dressing briefly if this occurs, then reapply and observe closely.

For Flail Chest: Stabilize chest wall with sandbags and ventilate with positive pressure respirator.

For Ventricular Rupture or Great Vessel Injury: Transport immediately; initiate massive volume replacement and aggressive antishock measures enroute.

Special Note

- Do not delay at the scene; expedite the run and transport as quickly as possible.

Transport

- Monitor patient very closely enroute, especially respiratory status.

CHILD ABUSE

Child abuse is said to exist when a child receives physical injuries at the hands of an adult, usually a parent or friend of the parent. Child abuse should be suspected in any situation where the injuries don't seem to fit the explanation given. Specific criteria for suspicion of child abuse include:

- history of repeated injuries, and/or delay in seeking care
- multiple bruises in various stages of healing
- cigarette or other burns
- belt marks
- injuries that are blamed on others, particularly siblings
- an alleged self-injury of an infant or very small child
- injuries in several different parts of the body

Perform a comprehensive assessment of the child following a head-to-toe format. Treat the presenting injuries as you would any other form of trauma. Control the ABCs, start an IV if necessary, and bandage or splint wounds appropriately. Above all, ensure that the child is transported for further care and follow-up.

Be nonjudgemental in your dealings with the parents. Avoid arousing suspicion, as they may refuse to allow transport. On arrival at the ED, report your suspicions and supporting findings to the ED physician so that he/she can take follow-up action.

TREATMENT PROTOCOL: CHILD ABUSE

History

- Under what circumstances did the incident occur?
- What was the mechanism of injury?
- When did the injury occur?
- Does the patient have any underlying medical conditions?

Physical Exam

- Is the airway intact?
- Are respirations effective?
- Is there any major bleeding?
- What are the vital signs?
- What is the level of consciousness?
- What is the skin temperature, color, and moisture?
- What are the findings of the head-to-toe exam?

Differential Diagnosis

Injuries can be the result of accidental or intentional trauma. Do not attempt to differentiate in the field, as it may arouse parent's suspicion.

Treatment

1. Ensure airway, give oxygen, and ventilate if necessary.
2. Control active bleeding.
3. If patient is hypovolemic, start an IV of RL or NS; use a Volutrol and run to maintain blood pressure.
4. If IV volume replacement is insufficient to maintain blood pressure, consider antishock trousers and possibly dopamine or vasopressors.
5. Bandage wounds and splint as necessary.

Special Note

- Don't press for detailed history of the incident. Abused children rarely supply honest answers, and probing questions might arouse parent's suspicion.

Transport

- It is important that the child be transported for medical care and follow-up investigation of the incident.

CHRONIC OBSTRUCTIVE PULMONARY DISEASE

Chronic obstructive pulmonary disease (COPD) is a general phrase referring to any longstanding respiratory disorder which results in obstruction of gaseous exchange in the alveoli. The two most common disorders in the COPD category are emphysema and bronchitis.

Emphysema is caused by loss of elasticity within the alveoli, resulting in enlargement of the terminal air sacs. This loss of elasticity causes the smaller airways to collapse on expiration, thus trapping air in the alveoli and resulting in hypoxemia. The patient breathes through pursed lips in an effort to prevent collapse of the alveoli. Other signs and symptoms of advanced emphysema include emaciation, chronic fatigue, barrel chest, use of accessory muscles for respiration, prolonged expiratory phase, and cyanosis.

Chronic Bronchitis is an inflammation of the bronchial tree which results in abundant mucous production and a chronic cough. This disorder can be caused by pollution, dust, fumes, cigarette smoke, and/or viral or bacterial agents. Signs and symptoms include a productive cough (usually without fever), dyspnea, wheezes, rhonchi, a prolonged expiratory phase, and chronic cyanosis in the late stages. The bronchitic patient may have associated congestive heart failure due to chronic pulmonary hypertension.

Treatment of COPD

Field treatment of acute episodes of COPD is supportive, consisting primarily of low-flow oxygen, position of comfort, and reassurance.

Although this patient is in respiratory distress, the pathophysiology of COPD alters the usual course of treatment. In a healthy person, the respiratory drive comes from a high serum carbon dioxide level, but the COPD patient needs a low serum oxygen level for respiratory stimulus. For this reason, the administration of high-flow oxygen can be detrimental, as it can cause loss of the respiratory drive with resultant apnea.

COPD is often a complicating factor in patients who seek emergency help for unrelated medical conditions. Patients experiencing acute medical emergencies often require oxygen to manage their immediate illness. If the patient has underlying COPD, the oxygen should be started at a low flow rate (1–2 liters/minute) and increased cautiously only if the patient continues to show signs of hypoxia. If an increase in flow rate is needed to manage the immediate situation, be prepared to support ventilation in case the patient's own respiratory drive is lost.

If an acute episode of COPD is causing severe respiratory distress, start an IV of 5% D/W TKO and give Aminophylline. Monitor EKG and vital signs closely, and transport in a position of comfort—usually sitting up and forward.

TREATMENT PROTOCOL:
CHRONIC OBSTRUCTIVE PULMONARY DISEASE

History

- When did the problem start?
- What was the patient doing when the attack came on?
- Has this ever happened before?
- Is the patient having trouble getting air in or out?
- Does the patient have a history of lung disease?
- Has the patient had any recent respiratory infection?
- Is the patient on any medications?
- Did the patient take any medications today?
- What usually breaks the attack?
- Is there any pain; if so, is it related to respiration?
- Is there a cough; if so, is it productive?

Physical Exam

- What is the rate, depth, and quality of respirations?
- Are the respirations noisy?
- What is the level of consciousness?
- What is the skin color, temperature, and moisture?
- What are the vital signs?
- What lung sounds are heard on auscultation?
- What is the EKG rhythm?
- Are the neck veins distended?
- Is the patient using any accessory muscles to breathe?
- Does the patient have a barrel chest?
- Is there any peripheral edema?

Differential Diagnosis

- Differentiate between an acute episode of COPD, CHF, and other respiratory emergencies.

Treatment

1. Ensure airway, allow patient to assume position of comfort.
2. Give low-flow oxygen at 1–2 liters/minute.
3. Try to calm patient, be reassuring.
4. Start an IV of 5% D/W TKO.
5. If distress is severe, give Aminophylline 3–6 mg/kg in at least 20 ml via Volutrol over at least 20 minutes.

Special Note

- If respiratory status deteriorates despite 1–2 liters of oxygen, may increase flow rate gradually, but be prepared to assist ventilation.

Transport

- Allow patient to remain in position of comfort, usually upright or leaning forward with arms on pillow.

COLD INJURIES

The occurrence and severity of cold injuries will depend on the actual environmental temperature reading, conductive environmental factors, length of exposure, and patient's underlying physical condition. Individuals who are particularly prone to cold injuries include elderly people who live in poorly heated buildings, transients who have poor shelter during winter, participants in winter sports activities, and people who partake of alcohol in a cold environment. Additionally, near-drowning incidents are frequently accompanied by hypothermia.

Cold injuries fall into two distinct categories: 1) cold damage to localized body areas (frostbite); and 2) generalized body cooling (systemic hypothermia).

Frostbite

Frostbite progresses from superficial minor tissue damage to extensive injury as underlying structures freeze. The affected area will initially appear red and inflamed, and the patient may experience stinging or burning. The tissues will then turn gray, white, or mottled, and the patient may complain of "pins and needles." As the tissues freeze they become white, waxy, stiff and hard, and the patient loses all sensation in the area.

Field treatment consists of protecting the injured area from further damage and gently rewarming the affected part(s). Do not rub or massage injured tissues, as this can cause further damage. As the part is rewarmed, sensation will return to the area and the patient may experience a great deal of pain. If necessary, morphine in small increments might be appropriate. Once the affected part is rewarmed, do not allow it to cool again; don't start rewarming if you won't be able to keep the part warm. Evaluate circulatory status of the affected part at frequent intervals.

Systemic Hypothermia

As the patient is exposed to continuing external cold, the body attempts to compensate by peripheral vasoconstriction and generalized shivering. The patient may experience listlessness, apathy, and sleepiness. When the core temperature drops to about 94°F, the body's normal regulatory system begins to falter, resulting in depressed respirations, hypoxia, and decreasing level of consciousness. By the time the temperature reaches 86°F, the vital signs are severely impaired, the blood pressure may be unobtainable, heart sounds might be inaudible, and the patient may suffer cardiac arrhythmias. Although 74°F is considered about the lower limit of survival, it is recognized that hypothermia contributes to a prolonged period of potential resuscitation; the brain can survive without perfusion in this state for more than 10 minutes. This mandates aggressive and persistent resuscitative efforts, even in patients who have been "down" for an otherwise unacceptable length of time, and who might appear to have no chance of survival.

Field treatment of systemic hypothermia begins with an immediate change of environment, removal of wet/cold clothing, and drying of wet skin and hair. This patient needs aggressive rewarming. Use blankets and, if you have them, hot packs or heaters. Immediate transport is indicated since the body can't respond clinically until core temperature improves. Enroute start an IV of 5% D/W TKO, monitor EKG and treat presenting arrhythmias, and support vital body functions as necessary.

TREATMENT PROTOCOL: COLD INJURIES

History

- What was the extent of the offending environment (actual temperature, wet or dry, wind velocities, other conductive factors)?
- What was the length of exposure to the cold?
- What precipitated the incident (alcohol, overdose, fall, etc.)?
- Does the patient have any underlying medical conditions?
- Was any treatment begun prior to arrival of the paramedics?

Physical Exam

- Are the patient's respirations adequate?
- How effective is peripheral circulation?
- What is the patient's level of consciousness?
- Is there any indication of frostbite; if so, what do the affected areas look like (mottled, red, pale, blistered, etc.)?
- What sensation does the patient have in areas of localized tissue damage?
- What is the patient's body temperature?
- What are the other vital signs?
- What does the EKG show?

Differential Diagnosis

- Rule out contributing factors such as alcohol, overdose, underlying medical condition.

Treatment

For Frostbite
1. Remove patient from offending environment.
2. Ensure patent airway and administer oxygen; assist ventilations if necessary.

3. Remove wet clothing; dry patient.
4. Institute gentle rewarming of affected parts, using blankets or hot packs; do not rub injured area or apply heat directly to the skin.
5. Apply dressings to injured tissues; protect affected parts from unnecessary movement or further injury.
6. If pain is severe, may require morphine sulfate IV or IM in 2–5 mg increments.

For Systemic Hypothermia

1. Remove patient to warm environment.
2. Ensure patent airway and administer high-flow oxygen; assist ventilations as needed.
3. Remove wet clothing; dry patient.
4. Rewarm patient as rapidly as possible; use blankets, hot packs, and/or heaters.
5. Start an IV of 5% D/W TKO.
6. Monitor EKG and treat arrhythmias (according to separate protocol).
7. Support vital functions as needed.

Special Note

- Once re-warming has begun, do not allow frostbitten areas to become cold again.
- If patient arrests from profound hypothermia, the time of biological death may be extended to 10 minutes or more due to the slower metabolic rate.

Pediatric Note

Pediatric dosage:
Morphine Sulfate: 0.1–0.2 mg/kg IV push over 3–5 minutes, titrated to effect

Transport

- Transport systemic hypothermia patients as rapidly as possible. Rewarming is the foremost priority, since other problems won't respond to treatment until core temperature improves.
- If patient is stable, no need for "red lights and siren" transport.

COMA OF UNKNOWN ORIGIN

Coma is a state of unconsciousness in which the patient cannot be aroused, even by strong external stimuli. It can be a manifestation of any number of pathological states, including cardiac/respiratory arrest, drug overdose, head injury, poisoning, diabetes, drowning, alcohol ingestion, or hypovolemia.

Your approach to a coma patient should begin with assessment. First, establish that the airway is open and the patient is breathing adequately. Check pulses, blood pressure, and EKG to assess cardiovascular status. Next, determine level of consciousness. Evaluate patient response to voice, touch, and deep pain stimuli. Determine whether the response is purposeful, or if there is a neurological abnormality such as decerebration. Check pupils to see if they are equal and reactive to light. Look for clues on the patient or in the environment that might point to the cause of the coma.

Since coma is so generic in nature, it is necessary to identify its cause before definitive care can begin. In the hospital, this will include exhaustive studies. But in the field, any extended attempt at differential diagnosis will delay transport and thus jeopardize the patient. Field treatment is therefore limited to supportive measures such as an IV of 5% D/W TKO and close monitoring of airway, vital signs, and EKG.

Some clinical disorders cause coma with such frequency that they warrant limited differential diagnosis in the field. The two most common disorders in this category are diabetes and drug overdose. For these conditions, it might be useful to give Narcan or 50% dextrose to elicit a response. However, if these are not immediately successful, don't waste time with other diagnostic activities. Simply stabilize the patient and transport.

TREATMENT PROTOCOL: COMA OF UNKNOWN ORIGIN

History

- How long has the patient been unconscious?
- What occurred immediately before the patient lost consciousness?
- Is there any evidence of trauma, drug/alcohol ingestion, or gas inhalation?
- Does the patient have a history of diabetes?

- Is there a Medic-Alert tag or wallet card, or any other pertinent medical history?
- Are there any environmental clues?

Physical Exam

- What is the respiratory rate, rhythm, and effectiveness?
- Are there any peripheral pulses?
- What is the level of consciousness?
- What is the skin color, temperature, and moisture?
- What are the vital signs?
- What does the EKG show?
- What lung sounds are heard on auscultation?
- What are the pupils like?
- Is there an odor on the patient's breath?
- Are there any signs of trauma, needle tracks, or bites?
- Was the patient incontinent of urine or stool?

Differential Diagnosis

- Rule out cardiac and respiratory arrest.
- The two conditions that commonly cause coma and are readily reversed in the field are drug overdose and hypoglycemia.
- Countless other conditions can cause coma, including trauma, neurological disorders such as CVA and seizures, poisoning, drowning, alcohol ingestion, and hypovolemia.

Treatment

1. Assure airway while keeping spine immobilized; suction as needed.
2. Give high-flow oxygen and ventilate if necessary.
3. Control active bleeding; perform CPR as needed.
4. Perform venipuncture for later analysis of baseline blood sugar level.
5. Start an IV of 5% D/W TKO; if hypovolemia is suspected, start RL or NS and run to maintain blood pressure.
6. Give Narcan 0.4–0.8 mg IV push or IM; may repeat.

7. Administer 50% dextrose 25 Gm IV push; may repeat.
8. Treat any associated injuries.
9. If patient doesn't respond, immobilize the spine, give supportive care, and transport immediately.

Special Note

- Utilize environmental clues to direct specific therapy, but do not waste time trying to diagnose in the field.

Pediatric Note

Coma in a child should suggest poisoning, diabetes, child abuse, or neurological disorders.
Pediatric dosages:
- Narcan: 0.01 mg/kg/dose IV push or IM; may repeat
- 50% Dextrose: 1 ml/kg slow IV push; may repeat

Transport

- Maintain close monitoring and airway support during transport.
- No need for "red lights and siren" transport if patient is stabilized.

DIABETES

Diabetes is a relative imbalance between body sugar and insulin levels, resulting in cellular deprivation of glucose. All body cells need sugar for metabolism; without it, tissues will die. A few central organs, especially the brain, have a more acute need for sugar and will die very quickly if deprived of it. Sugar is usually obtained from foods, and is distributed to the tissues via the blood stream. Insulin, a hormone normally produced in the pancreas, enables the glucose to leave the bloodstream and cross over the cell wall to be used by the cell. This process can be upset in one of two ways: 1) lack of sugar causes the blood sugar level to drop, resulting in hypoglycemia; or 2) lack of insulin prevents the glucose from crossing over the cell wall, so it remains in the blood stream and results in hyperglycemia.

Hypoglycemia (Insulin Shock)

The most critical of the two diabetic extremes is hypoglycemia, since sugar is needed immediately to keep the brain alive. This condition may occur if patients eat less than their usual diet, increase their activities abruptly, suffer from injury or febrile illness, or accidentally take too much insulin. Such patients appear to have fainted, or feel very weak, and exhibit cool moist skin. Vital signs are relatively normal. If the patient is alert, he/she will be extremely nervous, or may be unconscious or even experience seizures. Hypoglycemia often causes transient personality changes; patients may appear hostile aggressive, or exhibit bizarre behavior. This can cause patients to be mistakenly labeled drunk when they are really hypoglycemic.

Hyperglycemia (Diabetic Ketoacidosis)

In contrast, hyperglycemia has a slower onset of symptoms but the patient appears very ill. This condition can be caused by inadequate production of natural insulin, by skipping an insulin dose, or by eating an unusually large amount of food. Patients might have hot flushed skin, fruity-smelling breath, rapid weak pulse, low blood pressure, signs of dehydration, and may present with deep Kussmaul respirations. If patients are alert, they may complain of extreme thirst.

These are the two extremes of imbalance in diabetes, but a patient can experience any stage between them. Both hyperglycemia and hypoglycemia have identifying characteristics, but some of the symptoms are vague, they can overlap one another, and they are many times indistinguishable. The comparison of symptoms is shown in Table 1.1. It is frequently difficult to differentiate accurately between hyperglycemia and hypoglycemia in the field, particularly if the patient is unconscious. Regardless of which imbalance is present, a generalized field treatment can be given if the specific state can't be identified.

Treating the Diabetic

To aid in diagnosing an unconscious patient as a diabetic you should search for Medic-Alert tags or cards on or about the patient. Check for oral hypoglycemic agents, insulin preparations, syringes, or urine-testing materials. Examine the patient for injection sites, usually on the anterior thigh or abdomen. If the patient is older or has had the disease for some

Table 1.1: Signs and Symptoms of Diabetic Imbalance

	HYPOGLYCEMIA (Insulin Shock)	HYPERGLYCEMIA (Diabetic Ketoacidosis, Diabetic Coma)
Onset	sudden onset	slow onset
General appearance/ behavior	transient personality changes; nervous, hostile, aggressive; bizarre behavior; can appear drunk	appears very ill; sunken eyes; can appear drunk
Level of consciousness	weak, dizzy, uncoordinated; may appear to have fainted; can be unconscious; can experience seizures	can be restless, confused; can be stuporous; can lose consciousness
Vital signs	normal blood pressure; weak, rapid pulse	normal or low blood pressure; weak, rapid pulse; possibly febrile
Skin	cool, moist; diaphoretic	warm, flushed; dry skin; dry mouth and mucous membranes; may have signs of dehydration
Breath/breathing	normal	fruity-smelling breath; odor of acetone on breath; Kussmaul respirations (deep, rapid, "air hunger")
Pain	headache	possible abdominal pain and tenderness; nausea/vomiting
Other	intense hunger	extreme thirst

time, the legs may show signs of poor circulation including amputation of digits or legs, and the eyes may be clouded by cataracts.

If the clinical signs don't distinctly identify the problem, or if the condition is determined to be hypoglycemia, the patient must be given sugar in the most appropriate form. You needn't worry about giving sugar to undiagnosed patients because it won't hurt those who need insulin, and it may be vital to the survival of those who need sugar.

In the diabetic patient who is still conscious and has a gag reflex, administer Glucola orally. If he/she is unconscious or losing consciousness, start an IV of RL, NS, or 5% D/W TKO, and follow it with a bolus of 50% dextrose IV push. Severe dehydration frequently accompanies hyperglycemia, so you may be ordered to begin volume replacement. For those patients who are unconscious, and in whom an IV is not possible, you can give Glucagon IM or SC. Always try to draw a blood sample for a baseline blood sugar level before giving any form of glucose.

As with other chronically ill patients, diabetics occasionally call for treatment and then don't want to be transported after being stabilized. Stress to these patients the importance of being reevaluated medically since they may require changes in their management. If they still refuse transport, refer them to their private physician and be sure to get a release form signed.

TREATMENT PROTOCOL: DIABETES

History

- What are the symptoms?
- When did the symptoms begin?
- Is the patient on oral hypoglycemic agents or other drugs; if so, what kind?
- When did the patient last take medication?
- When and what did the patient last eat?
- Did the patient lose consciousness, fall, or injure self?
- Was there any seizure activity?
- Is there any other medical history?
- Has the patient experienced any personality change or unusual behavior?

Physical Exam

- Is the airway patent?
- Are the respirations effective?
- What is the level of consciousness?
- What is the skin color, moisture, and temperature?
- What are the vital signs?
- What are the pupils like?
- What does the EKG show?
- Is there an odor to the breath?
- Does the patient have multiple injection sites? Amputations? Cataracts?

Differential Diagnosis

Might be confused with head trauma, alcohol or drug ingestion, aspirin overdose, hypovolemia, arrhythmias, seizure disorder, or behavioral disorder.

Treatment

1. Ensure airway and ventilate as needed.
2. Give oxygen.
3. Perform venipuncture for later analysis of baseline blood sugar level.
4. If patient is alert and has a gag reflex, give 75–100 Gm Glucola orally.
5. If patient is unconscious or has diminished gag reflex, start an IV of 5% D/W, RL, or NS TKO and give 25 Gm 50% dextrose IV push; may repeat if necessary.
6. If dehydration is suspected, start IV fluid volume replacement with NS or RL.
7. If unable to start an IV in a known diabetic with altered level of consciousness, may give 0.5–1 unit Glucagon IM or SC.
8. Treat any associated injuries.

Special Note

- It is not necessary to differentiate between hypoglycemia and hyperglycemia, because no distinction is made in the field treatment.

Pediatric Note

Pediatric dosages:
- 50% Dextrose: 1 ml/kg slow IV push
- Glucola: 10–100 Gm according to weight
- Glucagon: 50 mcg/kg IM or SC

DIVING ACCIDENTS

The two major types of scuba diving accidents are air embolism and decompression sickness. Both occur as a result of the effects of changing atmospheric pressure on inhaled gases. As a diver descends, the air in the lungs is subjected to greater pressures and takes up less space than it would on the surface. When the diver begins the ascent, the air expands again.

Air embolism occurs when the air in a diver's lung expands on ascent, but is trapped in the lungs, either because the breath is being held or because laryngospasm prevents exhalation. As the trapped air expands in the closed respiratory system, the alveoli rupture and allow air to escape into the mediastinum and pleural cavity, causing pneumothorax and subcutaneous emphysema. Air bubbles from the lung enter the pulmonary artery and travel to the brain, where they cause embolization of cerebral arteries.

Signs and symptoms of air embolism include standard signs of pneumothorax, as well as tightness in the chest, shortness of breath, frothy pink sputum from nose and mouth, and dyspnea. Cerebral manifestations include vertigo, limb parasthesia, hemiparesis, loss of consciousness, and convulsions. Onset of signs and symptoms is rapid, usually before the diver reaches the surface. This is a critical condition requiring immediate treatment. If possible, transport immediately directly to a recompression chamber. Maintain patient in a head-down, left lateral decubitus position during transport to prevent further embolization. Give high-concentration oxygen under positive pressure. Start an IV and monitor EKG enroute. If seizure activity is persistent or prolonged, consider Valium.

Decompression Sickness begins when gases, particularly nitrogen, dissolve in the blood stream during a dive. If the diver ascends slowly, the nitrogen is able to leave the blood stream without causing problems. However, if the ascent is too rapid or too vigorous, the nitrogen bubbles remain in the blood stream, expanding as the diver nears the surface. The signs and symptoms of decompression sickness can be categorized as follows:

"The Bends":	aches and pains in and around joints
"The Chokes":	pulmonary distress, including dyspnea and cough
"The Staggers":	CNS manifestations, including mental impairment, paralysis, visual disturbances, vertigo
Cutaneous:	erythema, mottling, edema, crepitation, itching, paresthesias
Shock:	neurogenic or hypovolemic (secondary to emboliation of minute vessels)

Decompression sickness does not normally produce symptoms immediately. Onset of symptoms can be delayed 30 minutes to 6 hours. Depending on the depth and duration of the dive, the patient may experience all of the symptoms or only a few. The only real treatment is recompression, mandating immediate transport to a recompression chamber. Transport in a head-down, left lateral decubitus position to prevent embolization. Start an IV enroute and give high-flow oxygen. Monitor EKG and respiratory status closely.

TREATMENT PROTOCOL: DIVING ACCIDENTS

History

- What were the depth, duration, and frequency of dives?
- Did the patient ascend too rapidly?
- When did the patient begin experiencing symptoms?
- Does the patient complain of headache, vertigo, visual disturbances, pain, paresthesia, or paralysis?
- Was there any seizure activity?
- Does the patient have any underlying medical history?

Physical Exam

- What is the rate, rhythm, and effectiveness of respirations?
- Is there any active bleeding?
- What is the level of consciousness?
- What lung sounds are heard on auscultation?
- Are there any pulmonary secretions?
- What are the vital signs?
- What does the EKG show?
- Is there any subcutaneous or mediastinal emphysema?
- Is the skin mottled, itching, or burning?
- What are the results of a neurological assessment?

Differential Diagnosis

- Don't spend time trying to differentiate between air embolism and decompression sickness; both require immediate recompression before other therapy will be effective.
- Consider the possibility of underlying medical causes such as CVA, MI, or hypoglycemia.

Treatment

1. Ensure airway while keeping spine immobilized; intubate patient if necessary.
2. Give high-concentration oxygen; ventilate with positive pressure ventilator if necessary.
3. Start an IV of 5% D/W TKO; if hypovolemia is present, run to maintain blood pressure.
4. If patient experiences prolonged or recurrent seizures, give Valium 2.5–20 mg IV push in 2.5 mg increments, titrated to control of seizure activity.
5. If patient suffers profound cardiovascular collapse, institute advanced life support measures, including antishock trousers, vasopressors/dopamine, and antiarrhythmic therapy.

Special Note

- If decompression sickness is not treated in the early stages, it will progress to more severe manifestations.
- Recompression is the only real treatment for these disorders.

Pediatric Note

- Scuba diving accidents rarely involve children due to the proportionately small number of young participants in this sport.
- Pediatric dosage of Valium is 0.25 mg/kg IV push over a 3-minute period; may repeat once after 15–30 minutes; don't use in neonates less than 30 days old.

Transport

- Transport patient in head-down, left lateral decubitus position to prevent embolization.
- Transport directly to recompression chamber if possible.

DROWNING (Near)

The pathophysiology of near-drowning is altered by the type of water in which the patient was immersed, and clinical condition will vary depending on whether the water was salt, fresh, clean, dirty, or chlorinated. However, none of these factors will affect prehospital management. Therefore, discussion of this syndrome can be simplified.

The major clinical problems found in the near-drowning patient are hypoxia and acidosis. These are attributed to the common occurrence of aspiration of water and/or vomitus into the lungs, and the subsequent compromised respiratory exchange. Generally, the status of a near-drowning patient will be affected by the length of time submerged, age, concurrent injuries, and previous medical condition.

Field Management of Asymptomatic Patients

Following recovery from the water, the asymptomatic patient may appear stable and deny any distress. However, the onset of hypoxia, cyanosis, pulmonary edema, and lung complications may appear minutes or hours later. For this reason it is essential that all near-drowning patients be watched closely and examined at a medical facility. Field treatment includes high-flow oxygen, a thorough exam for associated injuries, an IV of 5% D/W TKO, and monitoring of EKG.

Field Management of Symptomatic Patients

The symptomatic patient is most often in cardiac arrest and should be treated in much the same way as any other arrest situation. This would include CPR and prompt airway management with an EOA or endo-tracheal airway. Ventilation should be with high-concentration oxygen under pressure. An IV of 5% D/W TKO is necessary to ensure a line for medications such as sodium bicarbonate and antiarrhythmics. Dopamine or vasopressors may be necessary to support cardiovascular status.

When resuscitating a near-drowning victim, do not waste time trying to clear the lungs of water. Anticipate that the patient may vomit, and proceed to pass a nasogastric tube and position the patient to prevent additional aspiration.

Assess the patient for associated injuries. It is not uncommon for the near-drowning victim to have concurrent spinal cord or head injuries, so immediate stabilization is required even before removing the victim from the water. Consider the possibility that a medical condition might have caused the accident. Attempt to rule out MI, anaphylaxis from jellyfish or stingray injury, trauma, or pulmonary injury following a scuba diving accident.

Keep the patient warm and monitor closely for EKG or vital sign changes. Collect a specimen of the water and take it with you to the hospital for analysis. Continue respiratory and cardiovascular support.

TREATMENT PROTOCOL: DROWNING (Near)

History

- How long was the patient in the water?
- Was patient pulled from the surface or the bottom of the water?
- What was patient's condition when pulled from the water?
- How old is the patient?
- Are there any underlying medical problems?
- Are there any drugs or alcohol on board?
- What type of water was involved (salt, fresh, clean, dirty, hot, cold, chlorinated, etc.)?
- What care was administered prior to arrival of the paramedics?

Physical Exam

- What is the respiratory status?
- What is the cardiovascular status?

- What is the level of consciousness?
- What are the vital signs?
- What does the EKG show?
- Are there any abnormal lung sounds?
- Are there any associated injuries (especially spinal cord)?
- Did the patient vomit?
- Is the abdomen distended?

Differential Diagnosis

- Was there any underlying cause for the accident such as an MI, hypoglycemia, anaphylaxis, seizure, or trauma?
- Is air embolism or decompression sickness a possibility?

Treatment

1. Assure airway while keeping spine immobilized and assist ventilations with positive pressure.
2. Give high-concentration oxygen.
3. Control any severe bleeding.
4. Suction vomitus as needed.
5. Start an IV of 5% D/W TKO.
6. If symptomatic, give sodium bicarbonate 1 mEq/kg IV push initially; thereafter, give no more than half that dose every 10–15 minutes for duration of arrest.
7. Treat arrhythmias according to separate Protocol.
8. Keep patient warm.
9. Insert a nasogastric tube to decompress stomach.
10. Treat associated injuries.
11. Treat hypotension if present.

Special Note

- Bring a sample of the water to the hospital if possible.
- All near-drowning patients should receive high-flow oxygen and must be transported due to the possibility of delayed complications.

- Do not attempt to evacuate water from the lungs.
- If any possibility of a scuba diving accident, transport directly to a hyperbaric chamber.

Pediatric Note

- Pediatric dosage for sodium bicarbonate is 1–2 mEq/kg/dose.
- Pediatric patients are more resilient than adults, so do not discontinue resuscitation prematurely.

Transport

- Use "red lights and siren" for an unstable patient and continue treatment enroute.

HEAT EXPOSURE

Heat injuries occur when a person is exposed to hot climate or is working around thermal equipment for an extended length of time. It can result in a wide variety of symptoms ranging from surface injury to heat stroke. The surface trauma of heat exposure includes those symptoms commonly associated with sunburn. Along with reddened and blistered areas of skin, generalized manifestations are common, including fever, chills, and malaise. In addition to skin damage, the patient can suffer heat cramps, heat exhaustion, and/or heat stroke.

Heat Cramps

Heat cramps can be found with or without other symptoms of heat exposure. These are muscle cramps caused by salt loss following profuse sweating. The patient has a normal temperature and needs salt to rebalance body fluids. If the heat exposure is allowed to persist untreated, the patient will deteriorate to heat exhaustion and/or heat stroke. Treatment of minor heat exposure is supportive, but includes cooling measures, change of environment, and possible oral administration of salt-enriched fluids.

Heat Exhaustion

Extremes of heat exposure will result in heat exhaustion. The patient displays normal temperature, but with accompanying signs such as cramps, nausea, vomiting, thirst, and in extreme cases, shock. Dehydration should be corrected with an IV of RL or NS, and the patient should be cooled gently.

Heat Stroke

If allowed to continue, heat exhaustion will progress to heat stroke. This is a true medical emergency resulting from heat damage to the brain's temperature regulatory center. At this point, perspiration ceases and the body temperature rises causing hot, dry, flushed skin. The pulse is full, and the blood pressure may be low, normal, or high. Systemic signs include vertigo, headache, seizures, ataxia, vomiting, diarrhea, abdominal pain, and coma. Treatment must include rapid cooling measures and change of environment. In addition, an IV of RL or NS, oxygen, control of seizures, and supportive measures should be instituted as necessary. This patient should be closely monitored. Death can occur from either irreversible failure of the temperature regulator in the hypothalamus, or by heart failure from the increased workload.

TREATMENT PROTOCOL: HEAT EXPOSURE

History

- What environment was patient in (temperature, humidity)?
- How long was the patient in this environment?
- Does the patient have any pain?
- Does the patient have any vomiting or muscle cramps?
- Did the patient lose consciousness; if so, for how long?
- Did the patient have any seizures?
- Does the patient have any medical problems?
- Is the patient on any medications?

Physical Exam

- Is the patient in respiratory distress?
- What is the patient's level of consciousness?
- What is the skin color, temperature, and moisture?
- What are the vital signs?
- Does the patient have any signs of dehydration or shock?
- What is the EKG pattern?

Differential Diagnosis

- Differentiate between heat cramps, heat exhaustion, and heat stroke.
- Rule out anaphylaxis, hypoglycemia.

Treatment

1. Assure that airway is patent.
2. Administer high-flow oxygen and assist ventilations as necessary.
3. Move patient into cooler environment.
4. Remove excess clothing.
5. *For heat exhaustion*, cool patient gradually with lukewarm water; prevent shivering.
6. *For heat stroke*, institute rapid cooling measures.
   a. ice packs to major artery sites
   b. sponge patient with cold water
7. Start an IV of RL or NS and run to maintain blood pressure.
8. Assess vital signs.
9. Do not give patient any fluids orally.
10. If suspected heat stroke, be prepared for seizures. May administer Valium 2.5–20 mg IV push in 2.5 mg increments.

Special Note

- Heat stroke is a true field emergency and requires immediate intervention.

Pediatric Note

- Check fontanels for dehydration.
- Pediatric dose of Valium is 0.25 mg/kg IV push over 3 minutes.

Transport

- Continue cooling measures enroute.

HYPERTENSIVE CRISIS

Hypertensive crisis is a syndrome characterized by an acute rise in diastolic blood pressure beyond 150 mm Hg, which is accompanied by other signs and symptoms such as headache, visual disturbances, vomiting, chest pain and/or seizures.

Hypertensive crisis may also lead to more serious complications such as left ventricular failure, altered level of consciousness, aortic dissection, or intracranial hemorrhage. The actual cause of hypertensive crisis is unknown, but precipitating factors may include renal insufficiency (chronic or acute), atherosclerosis, arteriosclerosis, or toxemia of pregnancy.

Treatment is aimed at prompt lowering of the blood pressure. This is a true emergency and needs to be treated as quickly as possible. However, field treatment is limited, making prompt transport a priority. Administer high flow oxygen, start an IV of 5% D/W TKO and monitor the EKG. Position the patient in a high Fowler's position to relieve lung congestion and decrease the intracranial pressure. Treat the patient symptomatically. You may need to give Lasix IV push to reduce the cardiac workload. You may also need to give Valium to control prolonged or recurrent seizures. Morphine should *not* be given to lower the blood pressure because it can cause vasodilatation and subsequent increased cerebral pressure.

Try to prevent a profound drop in blood pressure since this patient is accustomed to high arterial pressure and a sudden lowering can result in a myocardial infarction or a CVA.

Transport the patient immediately, monitoring the blood pressure every five minutes, or more often if the patient's condition warrants it.

TREATMENT PROTOCOL: HYPERTENSIVE CRISIS

History

- Is there any previous history of hypertension? Heart failure? Renal dysfunction?
- Does the patient have a headache? Chest pain? Visual disturbances?
- Has the patient vomited?
- Is the patient taking any medications (especially cardiac or antihypertensive drugs?)
- Is the patient pregnant?

- Has there been any seizure activity associated with this episode?
- Has this problem ever happened before?

Physical Exam

- Is the airway intact?
- Are the respirations effective?
- What is the level of consciousness?
- What are the vital signs?
- What is the skin color, temperature and moisture?
- Is there any muscle weakness or paralysis?
- Is there distended neck veins or edema?
- What are the lung sounds on auscultation?
- What does the EKG show?

Differential Diagnosis

- Cerebrovascular accident
- Congestive heart failure/pulmonary edema
- Acute myocardial infarction
- Seizure disorder
- Overdose/poisoning

Treatment

1. Assure airway patency, give oxygen and ventilate if necessary.
2. Position the patient in a high Fowler's position.
3. Start an IV of 5% D/W TKO.
4. If evidence of left ventricular failure, administer Lasix 0.5 mg/kg IV push:
5. Give Valium 2.5–20 mg IV push to control any seizures

Special Note

- Do not drop the patient's blood pressure suddenly as this may cause an MI or CVA.
- Field treatment is limited so expedite the run.
- Keep the patient as calm as possible.

Transport

- Provide a quiet environment—do *not* use "red lights and siren."
- Monitor the patient's level of consciousness and blood pressure frequently in route.
- Transport patient in high-Fowler's position.

HYPERVENTILATION SYNDROME

Hyperventilation syndrome refers to a sudden onset of shallow, rapid respirations in response to an emotionally-charged incident. Hyperventilation can also be a symptom of significant organic disorder such as metabolic or endocrine disease. It is important to eliminate true medical emergencies as probable causes before assuming the hyperventilation episode is purely emotional in nature.

The patient experiencing an emotion-induced hyperventilation episode is usually found with rapid, shallow respirations, usually in the presence of others, and gives a history of some type of disturbance such as a family argument or other dispute. The rapid respiratory rate blows off an excessive amount of carbon dioxide, resulting in an acid/base imbalance. Resultant signs and symptoms usually center around light-headedness and tingling or numbness in the fingers and around the mouth. Other complaints may include tightness or pain in the chest and carpopedal spasms.

Field management begins with a thorough history and physical assessment to eliminate probable organic causes of the episode. Once the problem is determined to be primary emotion-induced hyperventilation, reassure the patient and remove the audience if possible. Then place a small paper bag over the patient's nose and mouth and have him/her slowly rebreathe the exhaled air from the bag. By rebreathing the exhaled carbon dioxide, the CO_2 level in the blood is returned to normal along with the acid/base balance. If the patient does not recover quickly, you should consider other causes of the syndrome. You might want to start an IV of 5% D/W TKO as a precaution, and monitor EKG and other vital signs. Transport the patient for further evaluation.

TREATMENT PROTOCOL: HYPERVENTILATION SYNDROME

History

- When did the problem start?
- What was the patient doing at the time of onset?

- Has this ever happened before?
- Is the patient having any light-headedness or tingling/numbness in fingers or toes or around the mouth?
- Does the patient have any history of cardiac, respiratory, metabolic, or neurological problems?
- Has the patient recently been exposed to any toxins, allergens, or other foreign substances?
- Is the patient having any pain?
- Is the patient under any emotional stress?
- Is the patient on any medications?

Physical Exam

- What is the rate, depth, and quality of respirations?
- Are there any abnormal respiratory sounds?
- What is the level of consciousness?
- What is the skin color, moisture, and temperature?
- What are the vital signs?
- What lung sounds are heard on auscultation?
- What is the EKG pattern?
- Are there ary carpopedal spasms?

Differential Diagnosis

- Be sure to eliminate organic causes before labeling it an emotional reaction.
- Clinical disorders that can present with hyperventilation include: aspirin overdose, diabetic ketoacidosis, neurological abnormality, asthma, and many other cardiopulmonary disorders.

Treatment

1. Reassure and try to calm patient.
2. Remove any observers or move patient to a private area.
3. Cover patient's nose and mouth with a small paper bag and have him/her breathe slowly to rebreathe own exhaled carbon dioxide.
4. If symptoms persist, start an IV 5% D/W TKO, monitor EKG, and transport for further medical evaluation.

Special Note

- When in doubt, assume the patient has an organic problem and treat symptomatically.

Transport

- If patient does not respond to treatment, should be evaluated at the hospital to determine causative disorder.

NEUROLOGICAL TRAUMA

Neurological emergencies generally present as disruptions in the normal motor or sensory capabilities of the brain and/or spinal column. It is important to perform an accurate and rapid neurological assessment to determine extent of central nervous system involvement, and to establish an initial baseline so that any changes can be identified during subsequent evaluations. The neurological assessment should include an evaluation of the following:

1. Are there any abnormal respiratory patterns?
2. What is the level of consciousness?
   - Can the patient open eyes on command?
   - If so, is he/she oriented to time, place, and person?
   - Does the patient respond to touch or to deep pain?
   - If so, is the response purposeful, inappropriate, or neurologically abnormal?
3. Are the pupils equal and reactive to light?
4. Can the patient move all extremities on command?
5. Are the hand grasps equal and normal in strength?
6. Is the strength of the legs equal and normal?

Neurological assessment should be performed frequently and any changes should be reported immediately.

Head Injury

The threat to life associated with head injuries is the sudden or insidious buildup of pressure within the skull as blood or fluid accumulates. This increase in intracranial pressure can result in displacement of the brain stem, causing rapid deterioration of the patient's condition. Signs and symptoms of increased intracranial pressure include:

- decreased level of consciousness
- hypertension
- bradycardia
- respiratory depression
- nonreactive pupil(s)

Head injuries such as fractures, concussions, or contusions may or may not be critical. The patient with major head trauma who is not compensating requires maintenance of ABCs and protection of the spinal column; then immediate transport with IV and supportive measures initiated enroute. Field treatment of less severe head injuries includes airway management with protection of spinal cord, high-flow oxygen, IV TKO, and frequent reassessment of patient status. As individual circumstances dictate, cerebral diuretics and/or steroids might be ordered. Do not give analgesics to a patient with head trauma. All patients with facial or head trauma should be suspected of having had a neck injury and should be securely immobilized before being moved.

Spinal Cord Injury

Spinal cord injuries can occur in conjunction with trauma to the face, head, or neck, or as a direct result of a penetrating wound. These injuries can be life-threatening if respiratory muscles are paralyzed, or if low-resistance shock results. At the very least, they can result in devastating paralysis which can affect all motor activity below the site of injury. Signs and symptoms of spinal cord injury include neck pain, paralysis, decreased sensation, or deformity. Initial treatment consists of airway and respiratory support while protecting the cord from further injury. Start an IV TKO and institute supportive measures depending on the severity and extent of the injury. Be prepared to assist ventilations in all patients with cervical spine injury, as respiratory arrest can occur. Prior to any movement, immobilize the head, neck, and spine. The possibility of spinal cord injury cannot be eliminated based solely on the absence of pain or the ability to move the neck.

TREATMENT PROTOCOL: NEUROLOGICAL TRAUMA

History

- When did the injury occur?
- What was the mechanism of injury?

- Was the patient ever unconscious; if so, was it immediate with the injury or was there a lucid interval?
- What was the patient doing prior to the accident?
- Is there any evidence of alcohol or drugs on board?
- Does the patient have any head, neck, back, or shoulder pain?

Physical Exam

- Are respirations compromised in any way?
- Is there any obvious bleeding?
- What is the level of consciousness?
- Is the patient oriented to time, place, and person?
- Are there any signs of shock?
- What are the vital signs?
- What is the skin temperature, moisture, and color?
- What are the pupils like?
- Is there any fluid and/or blood in the ears or nose?
- Is the patient able to move all extremities?
- Is there any decorticate or decerebrate posturing?

Differential Diagnosis

Other conditions which may mimic neurological trauma include:
- alcohol or drug ingestion
- post-ictal state
- diabetes
- cerebrovascular accident

Treatment

1. Ensure an airway while keeping spine immobilized; assist ventilations if necessary.
2. Give high-flow oxygen.
3. Suction airway as needed.
4. Control any severe bleeding.
5. Start an IV of RL or NS TKO; if hypovolemia is present, run to maintain blood pressure.
6. Apply antishock trousers; inflate if low-resistance shock occurs.

7. If low-resistance shock is present, give vasopressors or dopamine; titrate to blood pressure:
   a. Levophed 8 mg in 500 ml 5% D/W or NS (16 mcg/ml) IV drip
   b. Aramine 100 mg in 250 ml 5% D/W
   c. Dopamine 200 mg in 500 ml 5% D/W (400 mcg/ml) IV drip; begin with 2–5 mcg/kg/min
8. If signs of increased intracranial pressure occur, consider use of cerebral diuretics or steroids:
   a. Mannitol 200 mg/kg IV drip per Volutrol over 3–5 minutes;
   b. Decadron 10–20 mg IV push
9. Do not give analgesics.

Special Note

- All head injuries should be suspected of having associated spinal cord injury; immobilize all such cases before moving.
- Neurological trauma can cause low-resistance shock and require cardiovascular support.
- Unless hypovolemia is present, run IV at a TKO rate to avoid increasing intracranial pressure.

Pediatric Note

- Check for bulging fontanels.
- Pediatric dosages:

Mannitol:	Same as adult dose
Decadron:	0.08–0.3 mg/kg over a 24 hour period.
Levophed:	start at 0.1 mcg/kg/min IV drip; titrate to blood pressure.
Aramine:	50–100 mg in 250 ml 5% D/W; start at 0.4 mg/kg; titrate to blood pressure.
Dopamine:	2–10 mcg/kg/min IV drip, titrate to blood pressure.

Transport

- Do *not* delay in the field.
- If patient condition is deteriorating, transport immediately "red lights and siren" and institute treatment enroute.

OBSTETRICAL EMERGENCIES

One of the most important decisions to be made about childbirth in the field is whether there is sufficient time to transport before the infant delivers. Signs of imminent delivery include 1) regular contractions at 1- to 2-minute intervals lasting 45–60 seconds each; 2) a large amount of bloody show; 3) a feeling by the mother of having to bear down or have a bowel movement; 4) crowning; or 5) the mother stating that the baby is coming. If the contractions are short, infrequent, and at irregular intervals, there is probably time to transport.

Field Management of Normal Childbirth

Once the decision is made to deliver the infant on the scene, try to provide a sterile field. Wear sterile gloves and prep the perineum with Betadine or saline to help keep the delivery clean. Instruct the mother to bear down only during contractions, and to rest in between to conserve her energy. Guide the infant's head to prevent sudden popping out, which can cause lacerations of the perineum. *Never* forcibly hold the head back to prevent it from delivering. Once the head has delivered, suction the infant's nose and mouth immediately.

As the delivery proceeds, the baby will rotate and the shoulders will present. At this point, guide the head downward to facilitate delivery of the upper shoulder and then upward to deliver the bottom shoulder. The rest of the baby is then delivered with ease. A newborn is extremely slippery, so keep a firm grip on him/her. Once delivered, attend to the immediate needs of the newborn.

After the cord has stopped pulsating, clamp it 6–8 inches from the baby at two points 2 inches apart, and cut the cord between the clamps. Within 10–15 minutes after birth, the placenta should deliver. Suspect that the placenta has separated and its delivery is imminent when you see additional length of cord extending from the vagina in association with a sudden gush of blood.

Save the placenta in a container and take it to the hospital. If difficulty arises with delivery of the placenta, do not pull on the cord or reach into the vagina to try to remove it. It is not necessary for the placenta to deliver prior to transport. Transport mother and infant as soon as possible. Anticipate an IV order for RL or NS. Pitocin may be given post delivery to control excessive bleeding, but should never be given in the field before delivery of the placenta.

Complications of Childbirth

Umbilical cord wrapped around baby's neck is dangerous because the cord can become too tight and strangle the infant. The cord is usually loose enough for you to slip a couple of fingers around it and lift it over the infant's head. If this is impossible, clamping and cutting the cord before the baby is delivered might be the only solution.

Prolapsed cord occurs when the cord presents first in the birth canal. Then, with the force of each contraction, it is compressed by the first presenting part of the infant's body, thereby cutting off circulation to the infant. This is a true emergency, for if not corrected, the infant can die. Place the mother in Trendelenberg position with her hips elevated on a pillow. Don't attempt to push the cord back into the vagina. Insert a gloved hand into the vagina and gently manipulate the presenting part so that it no longer compresses the cord. Transport immediately, maintaining this position constantly enroute and until relieved by medical personnel at the hospital. Administer high-flow oxygen and watch for signs of fetal distress, including a drop in fetal heart rate and meconium-stained amniotic fluid. If either of these signs occurs, note the time and report it to the hospital.

Breech deliveries can be readily identified because a foot or buttock presents first as the infant comes out of the birth canal. Most breech deliveries are slow, so you may have time to transport. However, if you are required to deliver an infant in breech presentation, allow the birth to proceed passively to the waist. Once this occurs, don't pull, but gently rotate the baby to a face-down position so that the infant's back is against the mother's pubis. As the delivery proceeds, gently support the limbs by wrapping them in a towel. This will make the baby easier to hold, help keep him/her warm, and help prevent fractures. If, after 4–6 minutes, the head does not deliver, insert a gloved hand into the vagina and create an airway over the baby's face by forming a V with your index and middle fingers. While maintaining the infant's airway, instruct the mother to bear down and apply *gentle* traction on the upper torso of the infant to facilitate delivery of the head. If you are still unable to deliver the head, transport immediately while maintaining the baby's airway.

Multiple births are an unlikely but possible field occurrence. You must consider this possibility and stay with the mother following delivery of the first infant. Subsequent deliveries can take anywhere from a few minutes to several hours. Each delivery should proceed normally, but there is a higher incidence of difficulty with each delivery, so every effort should be made to transport the mother between births. Once the infant is delivered and the cord is clamped, it is not necessary to cut the cord until all subsequent infants are delivered. Very often, the infants in a multiple birth are premature or unusually small, and one or more may require resuscitation. Watch the mother closely, as postpartum hemorrhage is common after multiple births because the unterine muscle has been stretched excessively.

Care of the Newborn

Following birth, the infant should be suctioned vigorously and stimulated to cry. This can be done by slapping the bottoms of the feet or rubbing the back. Determine an Apgar score immediately, and again in 5 minutes (see Table 1.2). Resuscitate the baby if needed. Monitor respirations closely since newborns, especially premature or small infants, need to be stimulated to continue breathing. If resuscitation is required, use mouth-to-mouth breathing, taking oxygen into your mouth before breathing it into the infant. It is essential to keep the baby warm and dry. Watch closely enroute and let the hospital know you're coming so they can prepare for your arrival.

Complications of Pregnancy

Postpartum Hemorrhage is excessive vaginal bleeding following delivery of the infant. It can be caused by lack of uterine tone, lacerations, or a coagulation defect. Field management is aimed at stimulating the uterus to contract. This can be accomplished by massaging the fundus, putting the baby to breast, and/or adding Pitocin to the IV. Additionally, administer

Table 1.2   Determining Apgar Score

Criteria	Score		
	0	1	2
Color	blue; pale	body pink; extremities blue	all pink
Heart rate	absent	less than 100	greater than 100
Respirations	absent	irregular, slow	good, crying
Reflex response to nose catheter	none	grimace	sneeze, cough
Muscle tone	limp	some reflex of extremities	active

high-flow oxygen and monitor patient closely. If shock is present, consider antishock trousers, IV fluids for volume replacement, and other standard antishock measures. Transport promptly.

Toxemia of Pregnancy is a disease which occurs only during pregnancy, and usually in the last trimester. The early stage of toxemia is called pre-eclampsia, and is characterized by high blood pressure, nervousness, malaise, edema, and protein in the urine. In the field, you will probably only see the last stage, eclampsia, which is manifested by seizures and coma. Field treatment of eclampsia is essentially the same as treatment of any other type of seizure, except that care must be taken to protect the fetus as well as the mother. In addition to managing the airway and protecting the patient from injury, you should give high-flow oxygen when the seizure stops. The use of Valium should be reserved only for extreme cases of recurrent or prolonged seizures, as this drug will produce a potentially harmful depressant effect on the fetus. Transport any pregnant seizure patient quickly and maintain a quiet environment, since undue stimuli can precipitate additional seizure activity.

Vaginal bleeding during pregnancy can be caused by a variety of disorders, but is usually attributable to one of the following:

Abruptio placenta:	placenta separates prematurely from the wall of the uterus
Placenta previa:	placenta develops over all or part of the internal cervical opening
Ectopic pregnancy:	ovum implants and grows outside the uterus in either the fallopian tube, the ovary, or the abdomen
Spontaneous abortion:	pregnancy terminates before the twentieth week of gestation

Vaginal bleeding in the nonpregnant woman is most often caused by menstrual irregularities or problems with an unidentified pregnancy. Pelvic inflammatory disease (PID) is a bacterial infection of the female reproductive organs or pelvic cavity which can produce spotting, but more commonly presents with abdominal pain and fever.

The amount of vaginal bleeding depends on the specific causative disorder and its degree of severity. In addition to vaginal bleeding, the patient may have some abdominal pain or cramping, fever, or obvious signs of shock. Regardless of the cause of the bleeding, field treatment is symptomatic and correlated to severity of the patient's condition. Standard measures would include oxygen, IV RL or NS to maintain blood pressure, and prompt transport. Rarely, you may be required to institute extreme antishock measures, including antishock trousers and dopamine or vasopressors. No attempt should be made to pack the vagina; this will not control the hemorrhage and may cause harm.

TREATMENT PROTOCOL: OBSTETRICAL EMERGENCIES

History

- Which pregnancy is this?
- What is the due date?
- Has the mother had any trouble with previous pregnancies/deliveries?
- Has the mother had any trouble with this pregnancy?
- Have the membranes ruptured?
- Is the amniotic fluid meconium-stained or foul smelling?
- When did the contractions start?
- What is the frequency, regularity, and duration of the contractions?
- Has the patient had prenatal care; if so, by whom?
- Does the patient have any history of venereal disease?
- Does the patient have any underlying medical problems?
- Is the patient taking any medications?
- Does the patient have any pain other than the contractions?

Physical Exam

- Are the mother's respirations adequate?
- Is the baby crowning with contractions?
- Are any presenting parts visible in the birth canal; if so, which parts are presenting first?
- Is there any bloody show or frank bleeding?
- What is the mother's skin color, temperature, and moisture?
- What are the vital signs?
- Does the mother have any peripheral edema?

Differential Diagnosis

- Determine if the delivery is imminent or if there is time to transport.
- Consider possible complications such as breech delivery, multiple birth, prolapsed cord, placenta previa, abruptio placenta, or eclampsia.

Treatment

If there is no time to transport, proceed with the delivery:
1. Ensure mother's airway.
2. Administer oxygen.
3. Start an IV of RL or NS if time allows; run at a TKO rate.
4. Support mother and guide the delivery.
5. As soon as the head is delivered, suction baby's mouth and nose; allow delivery to continue normally.
6. After the baby is delivered, assess Apgar score at one-minute and at 5 minutes; if baby is in distress, resuscitate as needed.
7. Allow cord to stop pulsating; clamp and cut.
8. Dry baby and wrap in warm blanket; put baby to mother's breast.
9. Allow placenta to deliver; do not pull on cord.
10. Once placenta is delivered, control postpartum bleeding by massaging fundus; increase IV flow rate if indicated. If necessary, give Pitocin 10–20 units in 1000 ml RL or NS and titrate to control of hemorrhage. If shock is severe, consider antishock trousers and other standard antishock measures.

Special Note

- If birth is breech, allow infant to deliver to the waist without active assistance (give support only); once the legs and buttocks are delivered, the head can be assisted out. If head does not deliver within 4–6 minutes, insert a gloved hand into the vagina and create an airway for the infant.
- If the cord is wrapped around the infant's neck, slip the cord over the head and off the neck; may need to clamp and cut the cord if it is tightly wrapped.
- In case of prolapsed cord, place mother in Trendelenberg position with her hips elevated on pillows, insert a gloved hand into the vagina and gently push the presenting part off the cord. Transport "red lights and siren" while retaining this position, *do not* remove hand until relieved by hospital personnel.
- If the mother is eclamptic and having seizures, treat symptomatically and supportively. If seizures are recurrent or prolonged and mother's welfare is threatened, consider Valium 2.5–20 mg slow IV push in 2.5 mg increments over 1 minute. Use Valium cautiously, as it may cause respiratory depression in the

baby as well as the mother. Transport quickly, but keep environment dark and quiet; avoid "red lights and siren".

- For vaginal bleeding, start an IV or RL of NS and run it to maintain blood pressure. Place patient in shock position, keep her warm, and transport promptly. Do not use Pitocin. If shock is severe, may need to use antishock trousers and other standard antishock measures.

- Consider the possibility of pregnancy in any female who is of reproductive age and complains of vaginal bleeding or abdominal pain.

- Multiple births are an unusual but possible occurrence. Be aware of that possibility and stay with the mother following the first delivery.

Transport

- With any birth that is difficult or not progressing, transport if at all possible.
- Keep the baby warm at all times; monitor respirations closely.
- Reassess baby and mother frequently.

OVERDOSE

The overdose patient may be found in any one of several stages of distress ranging from asymptomatic or mildly affected to completely apneic, with or without cardiac arrest. The sequence of patient assessment does not change, although you may need to work more quickly due to the urgency of the situation.

Drug overdose can be caused by prescribed drugs, street drugs, or over-the-counter drugs, alone or in combination, and with or without the associated ingestion of alcohol. The severity of the patient's condition will depend on the type of agent(s), amount ingested, time since ingestion, occurrence of aspiration, preexisting medical conditions, and patient's age. People may overdose themselves deliberately because of job problems, marital discord, or loss of a cherished person or object, or they may overdose accidentally because of improper labeling of the container, poor vision, inadequate lighting, confusion regarding prescribed dosage, or by forgetting how much has already been taken. Regardless of how it occurred, the patient must be assessed and managed without delay.

Field Management of Overdose Patients

Initial assessment includes the ABCs and a determination of level of consciousness. Check for associated injuries, especially fractures or burns that can accompany overdose. Gather as much information as you can from the patient, bystanders, and the environment to identify the substance(s) used.

If the patient is *unconscious,* it is essential to support the airway by proper positioning and the use of airway adjuncts. These patients often vomit, so have suction ready. Assisted ventilation might be required; use an esophageal airway or endotracheal tube if the patient is apneic. However, an EOA is contraindicated if Narcan administration is expected to revive the patient rapidly. Once airway patency is ensured, check vital signs, EKG, lung sounds, and pupils.

Give high-flow oxygen, start an IV of 5% D/W TKO, and give Narcan. If the IV can't be established, the Narcan can be injected intramuscularly. Narcan might have to be given as many as 10–15 times to be effective. It has a shorter duration of action than the narcotics it inhibits, and thus the patient may again succumb to the effects of the narcotic as the Narcan wears off. For this reason, it is imperative that these patients be transported to the hospital and observed closely for several hours.

Narcan is only effective in reversing the effects of narcotics and opiate derivatives; it is not effective against other sedative agents, e.g., barbiturates. However, it is administered to any unconscious overdose patient because often a combination of drugs, which may include a narcotic, has been taken and the patient may be helped by this narcotic antagonist. Narcan is rapid acting and will elicit an immediate response. Very often a patient will become combative following its administration, so protect the IV line from disconnection. As a diagnostic measure, you might also try 50% Dextrose in an unconscious patient. If the patient has been apneic, sodium bicarbonate may be necessary.

If the patient is *conscious,* get a thorough history of the incident, including type of agent, amount taken, and time of ingestion. Take vital signs, listen to lung sounds, and monitor EKG. If the induction of vomiting is indicated and the patient has an active gag reflex, you might consider the administration of Syrup of Ipecac. This drug should not be given if the patient ingested a petroleum distillate or a caustic substance. Other contraindications to the use of Ipecac include drowsiness or decreasing level of consciousness. If none of these contraindications exists, administer Ipecac and follow it with 8–16 ounces of water or other clear fluid. Position the patient to prevent aspiration and provide a receptacle for the emesis.

Street Drugs

Overdose from street drugs can occur when drugs are cut carelessly, a new batch of unproven strength arrives, or when the new user is experimenting. The chronic abuser is more street-wise but may succumb to an overdose due to generally poor health. Most overdoses result in seizures, unconsciousness, and apnea. When hallucinatory drugs like PCP (Angel Dust, Superweed) are taken, bizarre behavior ranging from paranoia to aggressiveness may result. These overdoses are treated symptomatically as no specific antagonist exists for hallucinatory drugs. Monitor EKG carefully, start an IV TKO if possible, and give Narcan to counteract any respiratory depression. Valium is used to manage continuous or recurrent seizures. Aggressive or combative behavior may necessitate restraints to protect both patient and rescuers. If the patient stares dully ahead, close the eyes and pad them. Avoid stimulation by keeping lights low, talking quietly, and avoiding using "red lights and siren."

Be honest, gentle, and nonjudgemental in your handling of the overdose patient. Explain the importance of proper medical evaluation and management. Protect the airway closely during transport, particularly if the patient has received Ipecac. Take all medication samples with you to the hospital, as well as an emesis sample if the patient vomited.

TREATMENT PROTOCOL: OVERDOSE

History

- What did the patient take?
- Did the patient mix any substances?
- How much did the patient take?
- When was the agent injected/ingested?
- When did the symptoms start?
- If unconscious, how long has he/she been unconscious?
- Has this occurred before?
- Did the patient vomit?
- Did the patient have a seizure?
- Had the patient been drinking?
- Has the patient had any medical problems?
- Is the patient on any prescribed medication?

Physical Exam

- What is the respiratory status?
- Is there obvious trauma or bleeding?
- What is the level of consciousness?
- What is the skin temperature, color, and moisture?
- What are the vital signs?

- What are the pupils like?
- What does the EKG monitor show?
- What are the lung sounds?
- Are there any track marks?
- Is there any odor to the breath?

Differential Diagnosis

Rule out:
- diabetes
- cardiovascular problem
- anaphylaxis
- trauma
- asphyxiation

Treatment

1. Assure the airway, ventilate as needed, and administer high-flow oxygen.
2. If patient is alert and has an active gag reflex, give Syrup of Ipecac 30 ml orally, followed by 8–16 ounces of water or clear fluids.
3. Establish an IV of 5% D/W TKO.
4. If patient is unconscious or has respiratory depression, administer Narcan 0.4–0.8 mg IV push or IM; may repeat as many as 10 times to elicit response.
5. If patient has been apneic, administer sodium bicarbonate 1 mEq/kg initially, and no more than half this dose every 10–15 minutes of continued arrest.
6. Give 25 gm 50% Dextrose to rule out hypoglycemia.
7. Suction as needed.
8. If patient has continuous or recurrent seizures, give Valium 2.5 mg IV push every minute, up to 20 mg, titrated to control of seizure activity.

Special Note

- Do not insert an EOA if Narcan is to be used.
- If patient vomits, bring sample to the hospital.

- Bring in all empty containers and syringes.
- May need to restrain combative patient to protect both patient and rescuers.

Pediatric Notes

Pediatric dosages:
- Ipecac: 15 ml orally, followed by 4–8 ounces of water
- Narcan: 0.01 mg/kg/dose IV push or IM; may repeat as necessary
- 50% Dextrose: 1 ml/kg slow IV push
- Sodium bicarbonate: 1–2 mEq/kg/dose
- Valium: 0.25 mg/kg IV push over 3 minutes

Transport

- Transport "red lights and siren" if patient status deteriorates.
- Observe patient closely for respiratory depression and/or decreasing level of consciousness.
- May have to repeat Narcan enroute.

POISONING

Poisoning is a very common field emergency that occurs in children 90% of the time. Countless substances have been known to cause poisoning in children, e.g., household cleaning products, plants, vitamins and minerals, aspirin, antihistamines, and cold medicines. Accidental poisoning in adults is usually caused by carbon monoxide gas, pesticides, chemicals, or drugs. Most adults who poison themselves intentionally do so with drugs or carbon monoxide.

Poisons can be ingested, inhaled, or absorbed through the skin. The effects on the patient will vary according to the substance's properties, the amount of substance contacted, the time since exposure, and the patient's age, size, and underlying medical state.

Local effects of poisonous substances can include erhythema, edema, tissue erosion, and pain. Systemic symptoms range from mild to life-threatening, and can include nausea/vomiting, weakness, confusion, seizures, unconsciousness, shortness of breath, respiratory depression, cardiac arrhythmias, and cardiac arrest.

Field Management

The paramedic's primary responsibilities in suspected poisoning are to:

1. ensure ABCs, establish level of consciousness, and check vital signs
2. support vital functions as needed
3. determine the general nature of the poisonous agent
4. take action to impede absorption of the substance
5. transport promptly

General guidelines for management of poisoning in both conscious and unconscious patients are shown in Figure 1.2.

Ingested Substances

For patients who have ingested a poisonous substance, you must first evaluate the level of consciousness and resuscitate if necessary. If the poisonous agent is known to be caustic or is a petroleum distillate, great care must be taken to prevent vomiting, which could create additional damage to the esophagus and oropharynx, or could cause pulmonary complications if aspiration occurs. Do not give anything to induce vomiting. Have the patient drink 6–8 oz. of milk, or water if milk is not available. Do not attempt to insert a nasogastric tube, as this can stimulate the gag reflex or could perforate a weakened esophagus. Give oxygen and transport as rapidly as possible.

If the agent is noncaustic and is not a petroleum distillate, and if the patient is alert and has a gag reflex, you can induce vomiting with Syrup of Ipecac. Take care to protect the airway, and allow the patient to remain upright enroute to the hospital. Do not give Ipecac if the patient is becoming drowsy.

Differential diagnosis of ingested substances can be time consuming or even impossible in the field, and relates to field treatment only on a superficial level. Specific treatment will be instituted according to Table 1.3.

Toxic Exposure Via the Skin

The patient's environment will often identify the causative agent in toxic exposures. As soon as a problem of this nature is suspected, protect yourself from exposure. This would include wearing gloves and keeping

---

*Reprinted with permission from *Emergency: The Journal of Emergency Services,* Carlsbad, California.

Field Treatment for Poisoning: Conscious Patient*

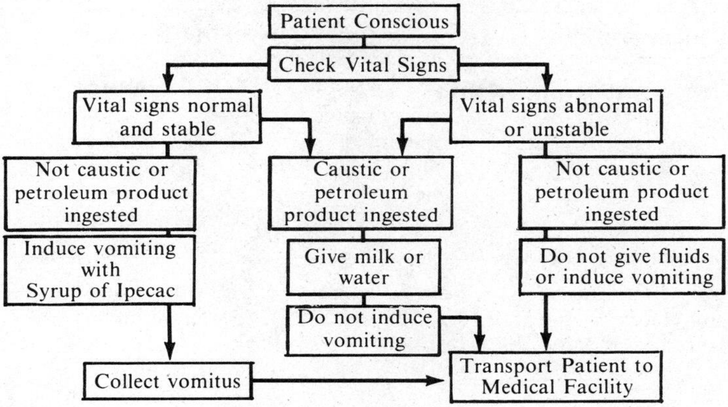

Field Treatment for Poisoning: Unconscious Patient*

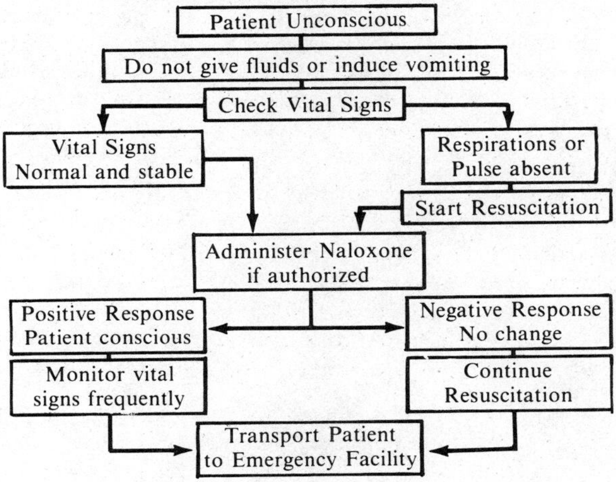

Figure 1.2. Field Treatment for Poisoning

Table 1.3. Field treatment for ingested poisons.

Condition of patient	Agent ingested	Field treatment
• Conscious; has a gag reflex; has stable vital signs	• Non-caustic and not a petroleum distillate	• Give Ipecac; give 6–8 oz. of water or clear beverage; protect airway; transport in an upright position
• Conscious; has a gag reflex; has stable vital signs	• Caustic agent • Petroleum distillate	• Do *not* induce vomiting; give 6–8 oz. milk (preferrably) or water; watch airway closely; give high flow oxygen; transport immediately
• Unconscious • Conscious with unstable vital signs; • Conscious without a gag reflex • Conscious but drowsy	• Narcotic, i.e., codeine, MS, demerol, heroine, paragoric, dilaudid, methadone, lomotil, percodan, darvon; • Unknown agent	• Do *not* induce vomiting; resuscitate if needed; protect airway, give oxygen; monitor EKG; start IV TKO; give Narcan; transport as soon as possible
• Unconscious; • Conscious with unstable vital signs • Conscious without gag reflex • Conscious but drowsy	• Nonnarcotic	• Do *not* induce vomiting; resuscitate if needed; protect airway; give oxygen, monitor EKG and respiratory status; start IV TKO; transport as soon as possible

the agent away from your clothes and body as much as possible. Quickly remove the patient from the toxic environment. Remove patient's clothing and wash him/her down with water to remove chemicals. If possible, use soap to clean the chemicals off. Evaluate vital signs and EKG, and support vital functions as necessary. It may be necessary to delay decontamination until the patient can be stabilized. A common surface toxin is pesticide containing an organophosphate base. Signs and symptoms of organophosphate poisoning usually begin within 30–60 minutes, and peak in two to eight hours. They include nausea/vomiting, increased salivation, sweating, diarrhea, tearing, visual disturbances, pinpoint pupils, slow pulse, muscle fasciculations, and eventually respiratory difficulty, pulmonary edema, convulsions, coma, and heart block. If the agent is an organophosphate insecticide, start an IV and administer atropine to reverse the parasympathetic effects of the agent. Transport as quickly as possible; monitor EKG and vital signs frequently enroute.

Toxic Inhalations

Protect yourself from the environment and move the patient to fresh air as soon as possible. Give high-flow oxygen and support respirations as needed. Monitor EKG, start an IV TKO, and watch closely enroute.

Home Remedies

Many home remedies and first aid cures have been taught on a large scale, but most have no documented medical value. In fact, they can be very dangerous, and some have been known to cause unnecessary deaths. Some of these "accepted" treatments for poisoning include emetics such as mustard powder, raw eggs, or water to which salt has been added. These remedies often fail to induce vomiting, and they can be detrimental to the patient or even cause death in some instances.

The universal antidote is a widely recognized remedy which has been shown to be ineffective. Another dangerous treatment commonly recommended is vinegar or citric acid to neutralize ingested alkalis such as drain cleaners. This does neutralize the agent, but in the process it generates an intense heat that is severe enough to produce thermal burns of the oropharynx and esophagus, thereby complicating the original injury. These procedures are dangerous and should never be practiced in the field.

If you have a regional Poison Information Center, you or the hospital can contact them to obtain additional information for emergency treatment.

General

Always try to bring with you to the hospital any containers or clues from the scene that will help the laboratory identify the toxic agent. If the patient vomits, bring a sample of the emesis to the hospital for analysis. Your primary concern is to avoid causing further harm to the patient during the treatment process. Monitor the patient closely, especially respiratory status, and transport as quickly as possible.

TREATMENT PROTOCOL: POISONING

History

- Was the poison ingested, inhaled, or absorbed through the skin?
- What did the patient take or come in contact with?
- If the substance was ingested, was it caustic or a petroleum distillate?
- Did the patient mix any substances?
- How much was taken?
- When did the patient take it?
- When did the symptoms begin?
- Did the patient vomit?
- What was the vomitus like?
- Is there any headache, dizziness, hallucination or visual disturbance?

Physical Exam

- What is the respiratory status?
- Is there any laryngeal edema, stridor, cyanosis, cough, or pulmonary congestion?
- Are there any blisters on the lips, in the mouth, or in the oropharynx?
- What is the patient's level of consciousness?
- What is the skin color, temperature, and moisture?
- What are the vital signs?

- Is there any parasympathetic effect such as increased salivation, tearing, urination, or bradycardia?
- Is there any muscle tremor or seizure activity?
- Is there any nausea, vomiting, or abdominal cramping?
- What is the EKG pattern?
- Is there an active gag reflex?

Differential Diagnosis

- Rule out hypoglycemia, neurological disorder, and allergic reaction.
- Distinguish between caustic and noncaustic ingestion.

Treatment

1. Ensure airway and assist ventilations if needed.
2. Suction as needed.
3. Give high-flow oxygen if symptoms are significant, support ventilations if necessary.
4. If symptoms are significant, start an IV of 5% D/W TKO.
5. Treat any arrhythmias or hypotension according to separate Protocols.
6. Transport as soon as possible.

For Caustic Ingestions

   a. Give milk, or water if milk is unavailable.
   b. Provide supportive measures and transport immediately.
   c. Do *not* induce vomiting; do *not* attempt to insert an N/G tube.

For Noncaustic Ingestions

   a. If patient is alert and has an active gag reflex, give Ipecac 30 ml orally, followed by 8–16 oz. water or clear fluids.
   b. If patient is drowsy, losing consciousness, or has a diminished gag reflex, withhold Ipecac and transport immediately.

For Organophosphate Poisoning

   a. Protect yourself from contact with the toxic agent.
   b. Remove patient's clothes and wash off toxic agent.
   c. Give atropine 2 mg IV push or IM; may repeat as needed.

Special Note

- Save any empty containers or samples and bring to the hospital.
- Rescuers should protect themselves from contact with toxic agents.
- If patient vomits, bring sample to the hospital.
- Watch patient's airway if Ipecac is used.
- Call Poison Center for specific directions if necessary.

Pediatric Note

Pediatric dosages:
- atropine: 0.05 mg/kg IV push or IM; may repeat.
- Ipecac: 15 ml orally, followed by 4–8 oz. water or clear liquids.

Accidental poisoning is extremely common in toddlers.

Transport

- "Red lights and siren" should be used if patient ingested a caustic substance or is deteriorating rapidly.

PULMONARY EDEMA

Pulmonary edema is an acute medical condition in which fluid gathers in the alveoli, thus impeding gaseous exchange. Several clinical disorders can present with pulmonary edema, including congestive heart failure, drowning, toxic inhalation, anaphylaxis, and IV fluid overload. Signs and symptoms of pulmonary edema include extreme apprehension, dyspnea, diaphoresis, cyanosis, and possibly distended neck veins. You may hear audible rales and rhonchi without the use of a stethoscope. The patient usually has copious frothy sputum, and it may be pink-tinged. The most common cause of acute pulmonary edema is congestive heart failure.

Congestive heart failure is a very common cause of pulmonary edema. It occurs when the heart loses its ability to eject blood effectively. Many patients who suffer MI, valvular disease, or hypertension are apt to experience varying degrees of mechanical heart failure at some stage of their disease. In right-sided heart failure, the inefficiency of the right chambers allows pressure to build up in the peripheral circulation, causing distended neck veins, peripheral edema, liver engorgement, and ascites. Other than its association with left ventricular failure, isolated right failure has minimal implication for the paramedic because it is not treated in the field. In left-sided CHF, blood volume increases on the left side, causing a backup of fluids into the pulmonary vasculature and the alveoli. Resultant signs and symptoms include restlessness, tachycardia, dyspnea, fatigue, orthopnea, dyspnea on exertion, paroxysmal nocturnal dyspnea, diaphoresis, rales, and rhonchi. CHF does not generally require emergency management unless it has progressed to frank pulmonary edema.

Field Treatment of Pulmonary Edema

Field treatment is aimed at relief of pulmonary engorgement and reoxygenation. Reassure these patients and allow them to remain in a comfortable position, usually sitting upright. Give high-concentration oxygen, preferably with a positive pressure ventilator to drive fluid out of the alveoli. If positive pressure ventilation is not possible, give high-flow oxygen per nasal prongs. Start an IV of 5% D/W TKO. Drug therapy begins with Lasix to reduce circulating volume, thereby decreasing venous return to the heart. Morphine sulfate is given to help alleviate anxiety and pool venous blood by peripheral vasodilatation. Aminophylline is used to decrease respiratory effort by dilating the bronchioles; it also decreases venous return because it acts as a vasodilator and a mild diuretic.

If the patient is in severe distress, rotating tourniquets may be applied in conjunction with drug therapy. They act to decrease venous return to the heart, thereby decreasing myocardial workload. When tourniquets are used, evaluate arterial pulses after each application and rotate systematically. Monitor the patient closely, watching for tachyarrhythmias and hypoxia-induced ectopy.

TREATMENT PROTOCOL: PULMONARY EDEMA

History

- What brought on the attack?
- Is the patient having trouble getting air in or out?
- Has this ever happened before?
- How severe is the dyspnea?
- When did it start?
- Is there any associated chest pain?

- Is there any history of cardiac or respiratory disease?
- Does the patient have respiratory difficulty on exertion or at night?
- Is the patient on any medications or special diet; if so, has the patient been following instructions?

Physical Exam

- Is the patient breathing effectively?
- Does the patient have noisy respirations?
- What is the level of consciousness?
- Does the patient have frothy pink sputum?
- What is the skin color, temperature, and moisture?
- What are the vital signs?
- What are the lung sounds?
- What is the EKG pattern?
- Does the patient have distended neck veins or peripheral edema?
- Is the patient using accessory muscles to breathe?

Differential Diagnosis

- Try to determine cause of pulmonary edema.

Treatment

1. Ensure patent airway; use positioning and suction to keep airway clear.
2. Ventilate with positive pressure ventilator if possible; if unable, give high-flow oxygen via nasal prongs.
3. Start an IV of 5% D/W TKO.
4. Initiate drug therapy:
   a. Lasix 0.5 mg/kg (usually 40 mg) slow IV push; may repeat.
   b. Morphine sulfate 2–5 mg IV push; may repeat every 5–30 minutes; titrated to effect.
   c. Aminophylline 3–6 mg/kg in at least 20 ml IV Volutrol over at least 20 minutes.
5. Consider rotating tourniquets.
6. Reassure and try to calm patient.
7. Treat arrhythmias as necessary.

Special Note

- Suctioning is often ineffective.
- Patients frequently respond promptly to drug therapy.

Transport

- Allow patient to remain in comfortable position, usually upright.
- Monitor closely during transport.

Treatment

1. Ensure patent airway; use positioning and suction to keep airway clear.
2. Ventilate with positive pressure ventilator if possible; if unable, give high-flow oxygen via nasal prongs.
3. Start an IV of 5% D/W TKO.
4. Initiate drug therapy:
   a. Lasix 0.5 mg/kg (usually 40 mg) slow IV push; may repeat.
   b. Morphine sulfate 2–5 mg IV push; may repeat every 5–30 minutes; titrated to effect.
   c. Aminophylline 3–6 mg/kg in at least 20 ml IV Volutrol over at least 20 minutes.
5. Consider rotating tourniquets.
6. Reassure and try to calm patient.
7. Treat arrhythmias as necessary.

RADIATION EXPOSURE

Exposure to radioactive materials is usually considered an obscure possibility, at best. In reality, however, the increasing use of radioactive substaces in all walks of life presents a growing likelihood that you will have to face a radiation accident at some point in your career. Old fears of nuclear war have been replaced in large part by more pressing concerns about laboratory accidents, fires in buildings where radioactive materials are used or stored, and the constant threat of transport mishaps by air, highway, rail or water carriers.

The severity of radiation exposure depends on the amount of body exposed, length of exposure, type of radiation, distance from the source, and amount of shielding. Time of onset of signs and symptoms varies also, but you probably won't see them for the first hour or two. Susceptibility to injury is greater in rapidly dividing cells, such as in infants and young children, and in the undifferentiated cells found in sex organs. Symptoms include malaise, fever, nausea, vomiting, and diarrhea.

Field Management of Radiation Incidents

A radiation accident presents concerns for both the patient's well-being and the safety of the rescuers. The following principles incorporate these concerns and provide a structure for safe and expeditious management of the radiation incident.

- *Evaluate Risk:* The first indicator that a radiation threat exists is usually the traditional yellow and black "Radioactive" sign. This can be found on the containers themselves, or on the building or vehicle housing the containers. The extent of the threat can be judged, at least initially, by the size of the containers. Generally speaking, a small container that could be carried by one person presents a small risk, whereas a larger container that would require two or more people to carry is probably "hot." Many fire departments carry Geiger counters to give a more accurate assessment of both the magnitude of the event, and the type of radiation being emitted. Finally, the driver of the vehicle or other personnel will usually carry a Bill of Lading describing the contents of the containers and the degree of risk.
- *Call for Specialists:* As soon as you recognize a radiation emergency, notify appropriate law enforcement agencies, as well as the local office of emergency services. An additional resource available to many areas is the Radiological Assistance Team (RAT) provided by the Atomic Energy Commission in areas of heavy radiologic traffic. This specialized team includes both medical and radiologic specialists who travel to the incident to assist with management and containment.
- *Minimize Personal Exposure:* If at all possible, use self-contained breathing apparatus. If this is not available, use dust mask or goggles to continue the rescue. Avoid breathing contaminated smoke; stay upwind of the incident. If the accident occurred indoors, shut connecting doors and turn off ventilating equipment.
- *Rescue the Patient and Stabilize Major Medical Problems:* Your initial emphasis should not be on the radiation injury, but on any associated injuries/illnesses such as burns, fractures, hypovolemia, etc. Most sources can agree that major injuries or acute medical conditions can be stabilized prior to decontamination without incurring undue risk to the rescuer.
- *Minimize Spread:* As soon as possible, clear the down-wind area. Patient decontamination should be attempted if patient condition per-

mits it. Radiation sickness is not contagious or infectious; one person can't catch it from another. But radiation particles can remain on the patient and be a source of exposure for the rescuer. Remove clothing and wash down with soap and water. Take care not to spread the contaminants to clean body parts. If the patient has open wounds, flush them vigorously with saline. If the patient has major injuries and can't be decontaminated, encase him/her in blankets to contain the radioactivity and transport to a designated medical facility. Be sure to notify the hospital enroute via radio. If the patient has only minor injuries, he/she should be segregated along with all other contaminated personnel, and held at the scene until released by radiation specialists.

Accidents Involving Nuclear Weapons

Nuclear weapons contain both radioactive plutonium and high explosives. When these weapons are involved in an accident, there is very little risk of nuclear explosion, but the non-nuclear explosives are a real concern. The plutonium can cause problems, but only if it enters the body by inhalation, ingestion or through the skin. With proper precautions, the threat to rescuers from plutonium is no more serious than the risk from the other products of combustion.

TREATMENT PROTOCOL: RADIATION EXPOSURE

History

- What type of radioactive material was involved?
- How far was the patient from the source?
- How long was the time of exposure?
- What type of shielding was employed?
- What types of injuries/illnesses are present in addition to the radiation exposure?
- When did the symptoms begin?

Physical Exam

- What is the respiratory rate, rhythm and effectiveness?
- Is there any active bleeding or other sign of trauma?

- Is the patient still in contact with contaminants?
- What are the vital signs?
- What is the level of consciousness?
- What lung sounds are heard on auscultation?

Differential Diagnosis

- Your initial emphasis should not be on the radiation injury, but on any associated injuries/illness such as burns or trauma.

Treatment

1. Evaluate risk.
2. Call for radiation specialists.
3. Minimize personal exposure using self-contained breathing apparatus; stay upwind of the incident; if indoors, shut connecting doors and turn off ventilation system.
4. Rescue patient and stabilize major medical problems; attend to ABCs prior to decontaminating patient.
5. Start an IV of RL or NS if trauma is involved.
6. Minimize spread: clear the down-wind area; decontaminate patient by removing clothing and washing with soap and water; flush open wounds vigorously with saline.

Special Note

- Radiation sickness is not contagious or infectious; one person cannot catch it from another. But radiation particles can remain on the patient and be a source of exposure for the rescuer.
- Contaminated patients with only minor injuries should be held at scene until released by radiation specialists.

Transport

- If patient cannot be decontaminated at scene, encase in blankets during transport to contain radioactivity; notify hospital to expect arrival.

Pediatric Note

- Young infants are more susceptible to radiation injury and present more challenge in diagnosing.

RAPE AND SEXUAL ASSAULT

Rape is defined as sexual intercourse (penile penetration) which is committed forcibly and without consent. Rape can be oral, anal, and/or vaginal, and can be perpetrated against both males and females of any age. The rape victim presents two distinct management challenges:

Physical injury is present in the majority of rape victims. It can consist of bites, lacerations, blunt trauma, stab wounds, strangulation, fractures, or mutilation. It can range in severity from mild to life-threatening.

Emotional trauma causing mental disorganization. This can present as confusion, disorientation, incoherence, and loss of time sequences. It may appear that the patient is presenting an inconsistent story. The patient's response to the acute shock state will present in one of two ways: *expressed style,* where anger, hostility, fear, and anxiety are openly displayed in the form of sobbing, crying, restlessness, and tension; or *controlled style,* where the patient appears outwardly calm and even uninvolved. Responses may be matter-of-fact or even seemingly inappropriate.

Field Management

Approach the rape victim with a calm, reassuring manner. Show the victim you care and help him/her legitimize feelings. Listen without being judgemental. Avoid asking about the incident; ask only about the patient's current condition. Avoid "why" questions, such as "Why did you let him into the house?". Try to have a supportive friend or family member stay with the patient.

The most common error made by emergency personnel when approaching the rape victim is to avoid interaction with the patient. This is a natural defense mechanism in times of crisis, and presents as appearing too busy, leaving the patient alone, and avoiding any emotional manifestation such as touching or holding. Be aware of this natural tendency, and try to overcome it by showing you care.

Limit your physical exam to assessment of major trauma. Do not examine the pelvic area unless severe bleeding is present. Don't ask patient to remove clothing unless necessary, and avoid any intervention that would further humiliate or upset the patient. Above all, explain everything you're doing before you do it. Talk to the patient about it, explain why it's necessary and how you will go about it. Go slowly and don't force treatment on the patient.

Field treatment will be limited to management of injuries in accordance with standard trauma protocols. Limit treatment to necessary care, and avoid delaying transport longer than necessary.

Special Considerations for Male Patients

Contrary to common belief, not all male rape victims are homosexuals. As with females, this crime is perpetrated on a wide variety of individuals, and is not confined to any particular group. The male rape victim will have many of the same problems as the female, except that the crime is usually much more violent. In the prehospital area, you will concentrate on trauma to the rectum, penis, mouth/oropharynx, and internal organs.

Special Considerations for Geriatric Patients

Elderly patients (over 50 years old) who are raped are usually subjected to severe physical injury, especially to the genital area. Physical force is used in 97% of all cases, and in 50% of them the patient is actually beaten. Rape of geriatric people is generally an aggressive act, rather than sexually exotic. It is also known to cause a permanent psychological impact, usually manifested by ongoing isolation and withdrawal.

Legal Issues

The rape victim has the right to decide whether or not to report the crime, and whether or not to pursue prosecution of the perpetrator. If the police are already on the scene, the victim can choose not to talk to them. Your role is to explain the pros and cons and then be supportive of the patient's eventual decision.

Unless the victim requests otherwise, you should do everything in your power to preserve any evidence of the assault. This requires that you discourage the victim from washing, cleaning up, brushing hair or teeth, changing clothing, using mouthwash, eating or drinking, taking any medications, or urinating or defecating. However, if the patient insists on performing any of these acts, you must respect those wishes.

TREATMENT PROTOCOL: RAPE AND SEXUAL ASSAULT

History

- When did the attack occur?
- Is there obvious trauma?
- Is there active bleeding?
- Does the patient have pain anywhere?
- How old is the patient?
- What is the patient's emotional state?

Physical Exam

- What is the respiratory status?
- What is the level of consciousness?
- Are there any signs of hypovolemia?
- What are the vital signs?
- Are there any bruises, lacerations, or fractures?

Differential Diagnosis

- Consider hypovolemia.
- Do not attempt to determine whether or not a rape occurred.

Treatment

1. Approach patient in a calm, reassuring, and non-judgemental way.
2. If physical injuries are significant, treat according to standard Trauma Protocol.
3. Avoid extensive or unnecessary questioning, examining, or treatment; do not delay transport.

Special Note

- Be supportive and show you care.
- Do not pursue questions about the incident; concentrate on the patient's current condition.

- Be very careful to explain everything you're doing; go slowly and don't force things on the patient.
- Preserve evidence if at all possible; if patient refuses, respect that request.

Pediatric Note

- Sexual assault on a child can involve sexual intercourse, *or* sexual stimulation of the child, *or* use of the child to sexually stimulate another person.
- Prior to examination, prepare child with an age-appropriate explanation of the procedure.
- Concentrate on the trauma aspects of the incident, rather than the details of the sexual molestation. Treat the patient as a trauma patient.

Transport

- Do not leave the patient alone at the emergency department. Stay with him/her until relieved by hospital staff.

SEIZURES

A seizure is the physical manifestation of disordered electrical activity in the brain. It usually presents as uncontrollable motor activity, but can consist soley of changes in psychological behavior, or it can be a combination of the two. A wide variety of medical disorders can cause seizure activity, including epilepsy, hypoglycemia, hypoxia, arrhythmias, poisoning, hyperthermia, and neurological injury. The significance of a seizure is determined by the situation in which it occurs and the type and length of the seizure activity.

Several types of seizures can be readily identified in the field. These include:

Grand Mal seizures, or general motor seizures, which consist of loss of consciousness, violent jerking of the total body musculature, rotation of the eyes, transient apnea followed by gasping respirations, flushing followed by cyanosis, increased salivation, clenching of the jaw with possible trauma to the tongue, and urinary and/or fecal incontinence.

Focal seizures, wherein the patient experiences alternating tonic/clonic muscular activity, but it is limited to an isolated body part.

These seizures frequently progress to involve larger body areas, and can mimic a Grand Mal seizure.

Petit Mal seizures are of very short duration and usually involve only changes in consciousness without associated muscular activity. These seizures are usually confined to children, and are so brief that they frequently go unnoticed.

Psychomotor seizures present as a dramatic change in personality, often manifested by sudden rage, hostility, or motor behavior inconsistent with previous behavior.

Hysterical seizures are a manifestation of emotional disturbance, rather than neurological disorder. They can mimic other types of seizures, but the patient rarely sustains personal injury or experiences incontinence.

The common phases of seizure activity are outlined below:

1. *Aura:* An aura is a specific, characteristic sensation preceding the episode and warning of its onset. There are many types of auras, including peculiar tastes, visual disturbances, auditory hallucinations, or imagined smells.

2. *Seizure:* The seizure itself is often composed of several stages as the seizure activity progresses.

3. *Post-Ictal State:* This is the stuporous state following the actual seizure, in which the patient can appear lethargic, somnolent, may yawn frequently, is confused or disoriented, and may complain of headache or sore muscles.

Assessment of Seizure Activity

Determine whether or not the patient has a history of seizure disorder, and if so, what pharmacological control has been attempted. It is also important to look for other possible causes of the episode, such as trauma, medical disorder, or toxic expsoure.

Observe the seizure activity carefully. Note its point of origin, time of onset, direction of progression, duration, and details of its appearance, including muscle groups involved, type of muscular activity, eye activity, and presence or absence of incontinence and tongue-biting. If you did not observe the seizure personally, attempt to get a detailed description from a reliable witness. Determine whether or not the episode was preceded by an aura, and whether more than one seizure was involved.

Treatment

Field treatment of the seizure itself consists primarily of maintaining a patent airway and protecting the patient from injury. It is common for patients to clench their jaws during a Grand Mal seizure and inadvertently bite their tongue. This is not only painful and potentially disfiguring, but can also cause bleeding and an immediate threat to the airway. If possible, prevent this complication by inserting a padded tongue blade or oral airway. Once the jaws are clamped, it is probably best to wait until the seizure subsides before attempting to insert an airway. Have suction ready to remove blood and/or excess saliva and position the patient for airway control and optimum protection of flailing extremities.

Cerebral oxygenation is of primary importance in these patients. High-flow oxygen should be administered immediately following the seizure. In seizures of unknown etiology, 50% dextrose can be given as a diagnostic maneuver.

Status Epilepticus presents a special management problem. It is evidenced by seizures that recur without an intervening period of consciousness. This prolonged seizure activity prevents adequate oxygenation, and the seizures must be controlled or serious neurological deficit will result. An IV of 5% D/W TKO is indicated, and Valium can be given to control seizure activity. Again, oxygenation is critical, as well as close monitoring of vital signs, EKG, and prompt transport.

TREATMENT PROTOCOL: SEIZURES

History

- Is the patient still seizing?
- When did the seizure start?
- What was the seizure like (motor involvement, progression, etc.)?
- How long did it last?
- Was there more than one seizure?
- Has this ever happened before?
- Does the patient have a diagnosed seizure disorder?
- Is the patient taking any anticonvulsant medications? If so, have they been taken as prescribed? Has the prescription been changed recently?
- Did the patient suffer any trauma prior to onset?
- Has the patient been exposed to any noxious substances?
- Does the patient have any underlying medical conditions?
- Is the patient pregnant?

Physical Exam

- What is the respiratory status?
- What is the patient's level of consciousness?
- Are there any lacerations of the tongue, head, or extremities?
- What is the skin color, temperature, and moisture?
- What are the vital signs?
- What are the pupils like?
- What does the EKG show?
- Are there any signs of paralysis, weakness, or unequal grips?
- Has the patient been incontinent?
- Does the patient have a Medic-Alert tag or wallet card?

Differential Diagnosis

Possible causes of seizure include epilepsy, hypoxia, cardiac arrhythmias, hypoglycemia, drug/alcohol withdrawal, poison/drug ingestion, meningitis/encephalitis, head injury, and hyperthermia.

Treatment

1. Ensure airway, give oxygen, and suction as needed.
2. Prevent patient from injuring self during seizure.
3. Consider 50% dextrose 25 GM IV push as a diagnostic measure.
4. For prolonged or recurrent seizures,
   a. Start an IV of 5% D/W TKO
   b. give Valium 2.5–20 mg IV push in 2.5 mg increments, titrated to control of seizure activity
5. Reassure patient.
6. Treat any resultant injuries.

Special Note

- Watch for respiratory depression if Valium is used.
- A patient in a post-ictal state may act lethargic, drift off to sleep, or experience short-term memory loss.
- Seizures in a pregnant woman may be an indication of toxemia.

Pediatric Note

- In children ages 1–4 years, seizures may occur with high temperature spikes.
- Febrile seizures should be treated enroute with gentle cooling measures.
- If seizures persist, give Valium 0.25 mg/kg IV push over 3 minutes.

Transport

- Watch for recurrence of seizure.
- Protect from injury.

SHOCK (Hypovolemic)

Shock can be generally defined as perfusion which is inadequate to maintain cellular metabolism. One of the major causes of shock is inadequate circulating blood volume; this category of shock is called hypovolemic shock. Although hypovolemic shock is most frequently caused by traumatic blood loss, it can also follow less obvious blood loss such as gastrointestinal or other internal bleeding. In addition to the hemorrhagic causes, extensive fluid loss can also precipitate hypovolemic shock. Examples of non-hemorrhagic conditions likely to result in hypovolemic shock include severe burns and extensive vomiting or diarrhea. A common cause of hypovolemic shock in infants and small children is dehydration.

Signs and symptoms of hypovolemic shock include restlessness, anxiety, mental sluggishness, cool clammy skin, pallor, tachycardia, rapid shallow respirations, thirst, and possibly hypotension. (Although hypotension eventually presents itself if the shock state persists, it may not be present initially due to compensatory vasoconstriction and tachycardia.)

Field treatment of hypovolemic shock consists of hemorrhage control, high-flow oxygen, elevation of the lower extremities (if not contraindicated), volume replacement with IV RL or NS, and inflation of antishock trousers in severe cases. If fluid replacement and the antishock trousers fail to stabilize the patient, dopamine or vasopressors may be indicated.

TREATMENT PROTOCOL: SHOCK
(Hypovolemic)

History

Is there any indication of trauma?
- When did it occur?
- What was the mechanism of injury?
- Does the patient have any pain?
- Where is the pain?
- Has the patient's level of consciousness changed since the incident?
- Is there obvious blood loss; if so, what is the estimated volume?

Does the patient have any current or recent medical problem?
- Has the patient been vomiting?
- Has the patient vomited blood or coffee-ground material?
- Has the patient had diarrhea or tarry/bloody stools?
- Has the patient been febrile?
- Does the patient have any pain; if so, what is it like?
- Does the patient have a past medical history of ulcers, cardiovascular disease, colitis, or hypertension?
- Is the patient on any medications?

Physical Exam

- Does the patient have any respiratory distress?
- Is there any active bleeding?
- What is the level of consciousness?
- What is the skin temperature, moisture, color, and turgor?
- What are the vital signs?
- Is there any unusual swelling or hematoma formation?
- Is the abdomen rigid?
- What is the EKG pattern?

Differential Diagnosis

- Rule out other types of shock (e.g., cardiogenic, low-resistance, anaphylactic).

Treatment

1. Ensure airway patency, give oxygen, and ventilate if necessary.
2. Control any obvious bleeding.
3. Start an IV of RL or NS and run it to maintain blood pressure.
4. If shock is severe, may require:
   - antishock trousers
   - dopamine or vasopressors after fluid replacement
5. Place patient in shock position if not contraindicated.
6. Treat associated injuries.

Pediatric Note

- Assess fontanels to determine hydration.
- Use a Volutrol to administer IV fluids.

Transport

- Transport as soon as possible; monitor EKG and VS enroute.
- If trauma is severe, provide minimal stabilizing treatment at scene and move to ambulance to continue treatment enroute.
- If trauma is severe, may transport directly to regional trauma center.

SMOKE / GAS INHALATION

The inhalation of noxious substances such as smoke or toxic gases creates a medical emergency by one or more of the following mechanisms:

- Asphyxiation: Oxygen exchange is prevented.
- Irritation: The substance itself causes damage to the lung tissue.
- Poisoning: The inhaled agent introduces a poisonous substance into the blood stream via the lungs.

Patients with inhalation injury can often be recognized when their chief complaint is respiratory difficulty and they are located near a source of gas, such as a chemical plant, heater, or fire. They may experience cough, pain on inspiration, depressed level of consciousness, seizures, and/or rigidity.

Carbon Monoxide Poisoning

Carbon monoxide (CO) poisoning should be suspected in all patients found unconscious at the scene of a fire, in a closed environment containing automobile exhaust fumes, or any patient burned in an enclosed area.

Patients with carbon monoxide poisoning often complain only of a throbbing headache coincidental with unusual giddiness. Other possible signs and symptoms include weakness, tingling in the extremities, confusion, reckless behavior, collapse, and coma.

Cyanosis can be masked because of the effect carbon monoxide has on the mucous membranes. The cherry-red coloring often attributed to CO poisoning is a late characteristic, and thus is an unreliable field sign.

Field Treatment

Although specific treatments have been developed for certain distinct gases, field treatment for all inhalation injuries remains basic. Immediately remove the patient from the source of the gas and support respirations while giving high-flow oxygen. It may be necessary to ventilate with positive pressure; in some cases, such as carbon monoxide poisoning, it is best to hyperventilate to help blow off the offending gas. Some inhaled irritants result in laryngeal edema, so advanced airway techniques such as endotracheal intubation or cricothyrotomy may be indicated. Do not administer any analgesics, as respiratory depression can develop. An IV of 5% D/W TKO may be ordered. Monitor EKG closely and transport as soon as possible.

TREATMENT PROTOCOL:
SMOKE / GAS INHALATION

History

- What did the patient inhale?
- Where was the patient found?
- Was the patient in an enclosed area?
- Were there any heaters, stoves, ovens, or fires at the scene?
- Was the patient using chemicals to clean?

- Was the patient ever unconscious; if so, what aroused him/her?
- Does the patient have a headache or other pain?
- Does the patient have any relevant medical history?
- Is the patient on any medications?

Physical Exam

- What is the patient's respiratory status?
- Are the respirations noisy?
- What are the lung sounds?
- What is the skin color, moisture, and temperature?
- Are there any singed nasal hairs or soot around the face?
- Are there any burns of the face or neck?
- What are the vital signs?
- What is the EKG rhythm?
- Are there any neurological findings such as twitching or seizure activity?

Differential Diagnosis

- Identify causative agent if possible.
- Consider neurological disorder such as intracranial bleeding, CVA, or seizure disorder.
- Rule out hypovolemic shock if burns are present.
- Do not overlook possibility of underlying medical disorder.

Treatment

1. Remove patient from harmful environment (ensure personal safety; wear breathing apparatus if indicated).
2. Ensure patient's airway; endotracheal intubation or cricothyrotomy may become necessary.
3. Administer 100% oxygen; assist ventilations if necessary; consider hyperventilating to blow off toxic gases.
4. Start an IV of 5% D/W TKO; may use RL or NS if volume replacement is needed.
5. If bronchospasm is present, may give Aminophylline 3–6 mg/kg in at least 20 ml 5% D/W via IV Volutrol over a minimum of 20 minutes.

Special Note

- Any patient found unconscious at the scene of a fire should be suspected of having CO poisoning and treated accordingly.

Pediatric Note

- Aminophylline should be used with caution in children.

Transport

- Use "red lights and siren" if either laryngeal edema or laryngospasm is present.

TRAUMA (MULTI-SYSTEM)

Trauma often involves more than one body system. When it does, it is considered life-threatening and requires immediate attention. Although the management of trauma is essentially a basic life support skill, the complexity of a multi-system trauma patient may cause you to move without thinking. To avoid this, keep the basic ABCs in mind and follow them in patient management. If you can control the ABCs you will probably be able to sustain the multiple trauma patient until the surgical team relieves you at the hospital.

Airway: Look for structural defects, such as fractured mandible, external trauma to the trachea, open chest wounds, or flail chest; intervene in any of these immediate problems. Check for obstruction caused by blood, bone or tooth fragments, or swelling; use suction and positioning to clear the airway. If appropriate, insert an esophageal obturator airway or endotracheal tube. Throughout initial examination of the airway, consider the possibility of spinal cord injury and keep cervical area immobile if at all possible.

Breathing: Determine adequacy of patient's respiratory efforts. Administer 100% oxygen and assist respirations if necessary. In a head trauma patient, hyperventilation might be indicated.

Bleeding: Rapidly survey the body and control major external bleeding.

Circulation: If circulation is absent, initiate CPR and standard resuscitative measures. Support blood pressure with IV volume replacement using NS or RL. Apply antishock trousers and inflate if necessary. Position patient to optimize perfusion. Monitor EKG and treat arrhythmias as necessary.

After managing initial priorities, transport as soon as possible. Immobilize the patient, bandage and splint injuries as required, and re-assess vital signs frequently. Do not give analgesics or oral fluids. Patients in this category will probably require the specialized care available at a regional trauma center.

TREATMENT PROTOCOL: TRAUMA (MULTI-SYSTEM)

History

- When did the injury occur?
- What was the mechanism of injury?
- Will extrication be required?
- Is there any blood loss; if so, what is the estimated volume?
- Does the patient have any pain; if so, where?
- Was the patient ever unconscious; if so, was it immediate with the injury or was there a lucid interval?
- Are there any underlying medical conditions?
- Has the patient ingested any alcohol or drugs?
- Is the patient on any medications?

Physical Exam

- Is there any trauma to the respiratory structure?
- Is the airway patent?
- Is the patient breathing independently; if so, are respirations effective?
- Is there any major controllable bleeding?
- Is circulation adequate?

- What are the vital signs?
- What is the skin temperature, moisture, and color?
- What does the EKG show?
- What is the level of consciousness?
- Is there any indication of neurological damage?
- What are the major injuries?

Differential Diagnosis

- Identify life-threatening injuries and set priorities according to the basic ABCs.
- Consider the possibility of underlying medical conditions that may have precipitated the accident.

Treatment

1. Ensure patent airway while keeping spine immobile; intubate if necessary.
2. Assist ventilations if necessary; use 100% oxygen.
3. Control active bleeding.
4. Start an IV of RL or NS using a large bore cannula needle; may need to start more than one IV.
5. Apply antishock trousers and inflate as necessary.
6. Keep patient warm.
7. Apply dressings as needed; splint any fractures; immobilize spine for transport.
8. Do not give any analgesics or oral fluids.

Special Note

- If fluid replacement and antishock trousers fail to maintain blood pressure, may try dopamine or vasopressors.
- If injury is isolated, such as a hand caught in machinery, may consider morphine sulfate in 2 mg increments IV push.

Pediatric Note

- Consider child abuse.

Transport

- *Do not delay in the field*. Transport as soon as possible, instituting treatment enroute.
- Patients with severe multi-system trauma should be transported directly to a regional trauma center.
- Stabilize all injuries before moving the patient.

VENOMOUS LAND ANIMALS

Snakebite

It has been estimated that in nearly 25% of all bites from poisonous snakes, *no* venom has been released, so you must first determine whether or not the snake actually injected venom with its bite. Indications that this has occurred include rapid onset (within 3–10 minutes) of pain, redness, and swelling at the site. The severity of response to envenomation is determined by the intensity of symptoms and how quickly they appear following the bite. These can be influenced by the size and type of the snake, the size of the patient, how much venom the snake injected, whether or not the bite penetrated the vascular system, and the general medical condition of the patient. Children will be more severely affected because of the proportionately large amount of venom injected.

Pit Vipers

The venom of pit vipers (including rattlesnakes, water moccasins, and copperheads) destroys red blood cells, interferes with coagulation, and destroys body tissues. When reporting to the hospital, it is important to differentiate between local and systemic symptoms, since these categories will be used to grade the severity of the reaction. Local symptoms include pain, redness, and swelling at the site. General systemic symptoms include sustained tachycardia and tachypnea, tingling around the mouth, shortness of breath, weakness, faintness, nausea, and muscle tremors. These can progress quickly to hematemesis, hematuria, respiratory depression, and coma. In extreme cases, death can occur within an hour.

As soon as you suspect envenomation, calm the patient, sit him/her down and do not allow movement; any movement at all will further circulate the venom. Place a constricting band just proximal to the site, adjusting it to occlude venous return, but ensuring that an arterial pulse is palpable in the extremity. Keep the affected limb below the level of the heart to delay absorption. If you arrive within 10 minutes after envenomation and the hospital is more than an hour away, you may be ordered to make two small incisions over the fang marks. These should be parallel to the extremity if possible, and about ⅛–¼ inch deep (down to the venom), and no more than about ¼ inch long. Apply suction and continue during transport.

Start an IV of 5% D/W TKO and watch respiratory and cardiovascular status closely. Analgesics are contraindicated for snakebites because they can aggravate some of the symptoms. Ice has long been used to slow circulation in the area and to help reduce pain. However, ice itself can cause tissue necrosis, and should only be used if wrapped in cloth to protect the tissues. Never soak the limb in ice water, as extensive damage can result. When you transport these patients, they must be carried to the ambulance; do not allow them to walk.

Coral Snakes

Another category of poisonous snakes is the coral snake group, whose highly toxic venom can cause death by paralysis if not treated immediately. As with pit vipers, the symptoms can range from mild to severe, and may be local or systemic. Systemic symptoms are primarily neurologic, and may not appear for as long as 18 hours after the bite.

Once it is established that envenomation has actually occurred, begin treatment promptly. Field treatment is the same as the treatment of pit viper injuries.

Spider Bites

The two spiders which most commonly cause problems are the Black Widow and the Brown Recluse, or Violin Spider. Bites of these spiders are usually identified by small, painful, red blebs associated with general symptoms ranging from gastrointestinal upset to anaphylaxis. A good history and physical exam will facilitate proper diagnosis. Specific antidotes are available for common poisonous bites, so prompt transport is indicated. During transport, monitor the patient closely and support vital body functions as required.

TREATMENT PROTOCOL: VENOMOUS LAND ANIMALS

History

- How long ago was the patient bitten?
- When did the symptoms first appear?
- Where on the patient is the bite located?
- What kind of snake/spider was it?
- Has the patient's level of consciousness changed since the incident?
- Was any treatment instituted prior to arrival of the paramedics?
- Does the patient have any shortness of breath, tingling around the mouth, abdominal cramps, chest pain, weakness, nausea, or muscle temors?
- Is there any underlying medical condition?

Physical Exam

- Is the patient having any respiratory distress?
- What is the level of consciousness?
- What does the surface wound look like (are there fang/bite marks, blebs, more than one bite, etc.)?
- Is there redness, swelling, or pain at the site?
- What are the vital signs?
- What is the skin temperature, color, and moisture?
- What is the EKG pattern?
- Are there any signs of systemic involvement?

Differential Diagnosis

- Must differentiate between local and systemic reaction.
- Try to determine type of venomous animal involved.
- Consider possibility of concurrent allergic reaction.

Treatment

1. Administer high-flow oxygen if patient is having respiratory distress.

2. Lay patient down and instruct him/her not to move unnecessarily.

3. Place a constricting band prominal to the site, if feasible, to occlude only venous return.

4. Keep area dependent to slow circulation of venom.

5. Apply cool pack to extremity; do *not* use ice in direct contact with skin; do *not* soak area in ice water.

6. Start an IV of 5% D/W TKO.

7. *For Snakebite:* If envenomation occurred less than 10 minutes ago and the hospital is more than an hour away, incise the site and apply continuous suction:

   a. incisions must be *small*, from 1/8 to 1/4 inch deep, and no more than 1/4 inch long

   b. incise directly over the fang marks, keeping the incisions parallel to the extremity if possible

Special Note

- Do not give analgesics.
- Try to bring snake/spider in for positive identification if this can be accomplished without risk to personal safety.
- Might administer conjunctival skin test for antivenin sensitivity prior to arrival at the hospital.
- If reaction is severe, patient may require cardiovascular support.

Pediatric Note

- Children will be more severely affected because of the proportionately large volume of venom injected.

Transport

- Transport promptly, as victim is in need of antivenin as soon as possible.

- Do not allow the patient to walk to the ambulance; must be carried to prevent unnecessary movement.
- All victims of venomous animal bite should be evaluated in the ED.

VENOMOUS WATER ANIMALS

Two of the more common categories of venomous water animals that can cause systemic symptoms and require advanced life support are stingrays and coelenterates.

Stingrays inhabit waters of the North American coast. They have spines located along the dorsum of their tails with which they wound victims who unwittingly step on them. The spines are surrounded by integumentary sheaths containing venom. When the spine punctures the victim's skin, usually on the foot or ankle, the venom is released from the sheath causing immediate, severe pain. The wound is usually a ragged cut with reddened edges, and may bleed freely. Vasovagal symptoms such as syncope, weakness, and nausea may also occur.

Portions of the sheath may be retained in the wound; if visible, they should be removed and any active bleeding controlled. The venom is heat labile, therefore, the injured area should be immersed in water as hot as the patient can tolerate. The heat will deactivate the venom and markedly relieve the pain. Observe the patient for systemic symptoms and treat accordingly. On rare occasions anaphylaxis has been reported.

Coelenterates such as jellyfish, corals, and sea anemones all have tentacles which contain hundreds of sting units capable of penetrating the skin. Envenomation occurs along the lines where the tentacles contact the skin. The areas contracted appear red and raised, and the patient will complain of pain and itching at the sites. Systemic signs and symptoms may occur, including weakness, nausea, headache, muscle pain and spasms, changes in pulse rate, and chest pain associated with respirations.

Some sting units on the skin may not initially inject their venom, but may be stimulated to do so with the application of pressure or changes in pH. Initial treatment, therefore, involves pouring alcohol over the involved area. This deactivates any sting units that remain intact. Once this is done, any remaining portions of tentacles can be safely removed with a gloved hand. Baking soda or meat tenderizer may help alleviate local symptoms. The baking soda should be applied as a paste to the affected areas and allowed to dry before scraping it off with a knife edge. This removes any deactivated sting units left embedded in the skin. Systemic symptoms, including anaphylaxis, should be treated supportively with oxygen, an IV of 5% D/W TKO, and appropriate drug therapy.

TREATMENT PROTOCOL: VENOMOUS WATER ANIMALS

History

- What kind of water animal came in contact with the patient?
- Is there any pain; if so, where is it and what is it like?
- When did the injury occur?
- When did the patient begin having symptoms?
- Does the patient have a history of allergies?
- Does the patient have any systemic symptoms such as nausea, palpitations, headache, syncope?

Physical Exam

- Is there any difficulty breathing?
- What is the level of consciousness?
- What are the lung sounds?
- What is the skin color, temperature, and moisture?
- Are there any lacerations, sting marks, welts, or hives?
- Is there any swelling; if so, is it localized or general?
- What are the vital signs?
- What is the EKG pattern?

Differential Diagnosis

- Identify the causative agent (type of marine animal).
- Distinguish between local and systemic reaction.

Treatment

1. Ensure airway, give oxygen, and assist ventilations if necessary.
2. *If Stingray Injury,* remove barb if possible; apply heat locally. Control bleeding and dress wound.
3. *If Jellyfish Injury,* rinse with alcohol; remove tentacles; apply baking soda paste or meat tenderizer to alleviate pain.

4. *If allergic response is developing,* apply constricting band proximal to the site if possible; give epinephrine 1:1,000 0.3 mg SC; may repeat 3 times at 5 minute intervals.
5. If necessary, start an IV of 5% D/W TKO.
6. Reassure patient; keep him/her calm.

Special Note

- If severe allergic reaction is developing, consider intubation.
- Do not give analgesics for pain.

Pediatric Note

Pediatric dosage of epinephrine is 0.01 mg/kg 1:1,000 SC; may repeat 3 times at 20 minute intervals to a maximum of 0.3 mg.

Transport

- No need for "red lights and siren" if patient is stabilized.

SELF-ASSESSMENT QUESTIONS

ACUTE ABDOMINAL PAIN 5

1. What is the most common cause of shock associated with acute abdominal pain?

2. What clinical disorder is suggested when you see a pulsating mass in the abdomen?

3. Why do you *not* palpate a pulsating abdominal mass?

4. Why is prompt transport indicated for patients with acute abdominal pain?

5. What is the clinical picture of a patient with abdominal pain?

6. What are the general principles for treating patients with abdominal pain?

7. What are the major contraindications in treatment of patients with acute abdominal pain?

ABDOMINAL TRAUMA 8

1. What are the two major categories of abdominal trauma?

2. What type of shock is commonly associated with abdominal trauma?

3. What clinical signs are associated with abdominal trauma?

4. What major assessment parameters should be included in your examination of the abdominal trauma patient?

5. What field treatment should be administered to an abdominal trauma patient?

6. What are the major contraindications in treatment of patients with abdominal trauma?

7. If the patient has a penetrating object protruding from the abdomen, how will this alter management?

AIRWAY OBSTRUCTION 10

1. What are the two major types of upper airway obstruction?

2. Why is airway obstruction a major emergency?

3. What are the most common causes of foreign body obstruction?

4. What types of clinical conditions will cause edema of the airways capable of obstructing respiration?

5. How do you differentiate between a partial airway obstruction and complete obstruction?

6. How would you treat a foreign body obstruction if the patient is conscious and able to talk?

7. How would you treat a foreign body obstruction if the patient is conscious but unable to talk or exchange air?

8. How would you treat a foreign body obstruction if the patient is unconscious when found or loses consciousness?

9. How would you treat obstruction due to laryngeal edema associated with anaphylaxis?

10. How would you treat obstruction due to laryngeal edema associated with respiratory burns?

11. How would you treat a child suspected of having croup or epiglottitis?

12. What management obligations do you have after the obstruction is relieved?

ALLERGIC REACTION / ANAPHYLAXIS 14

1. What role does histamine play in an allergic reaction?

2. How does an allergic reaction affect the bronchial tree? The peripheral blood vessels? Cell permeability?

3. What signs and symptoms are characteristic of allergic reaction/anaphylaxis?

4. What treatment principles are used to treat allergic reaction/anaphylaxis?

5. What action does epinephrine have in the treatment of acute allergic reaction/anaphylaxis?

6. What action does Benadryl have in the treatment of acute allergic reaction/anaphylaxis?

7. If the patient is suffering a severe anaphylactic reaction, and is hypotensive or experiencing respiratory difficulty, how might you modify your treatment?

ARRHYTHMIAS 17

1. In which clinical conditions might you anticipate arrhythmias?

2. What general procedures must be performed on all patients who are having arrhythmias or have the potential for them?

3. How do you know which arrhythmias to treat and which to watch?

4. What three categories of arrhythmias are known to produce symptoms of reduced cardiac output?

5. What are the signs/symptoms of drop in cardiac output?

6. How do you treat supraventricular tachyarrhythmias?

7. How do you treat supraventricular bradyarrhythmias?

8. How do you treat PVCs or ventricular tachycardia where the patient *is* perfusing?

9. How do you treat ventricular tachycardia where the patient is *not* perfusing?

10. How do you treat ventricular fibrillation?

11. How do you treat recurring or refractory ventricular fibrillation which does not respond to other measures?

12. How do you treat second or third degree heart blocks at the ventricular level, and idioventricular rhythm?

13. How do you treat asystole and electromechanical dissociation?

14. What role does sodium bicarbonate play in the treatment of arrhythmias? What is the dosage and how is it given?

15. Why must atropine be used cautiously in the presence of an MI?

16. What restrictions are placed on the use of a precordial thump?

ASTHMA   22

1. What are the signs/symptoms of an acute asthma attack?

2. What factors might have precipitated the attack?

3. How is the environment important in the management of an acute asthma attack?

4. What is the treatment regimen for acute asthma attack?

5. What other disorders might be confused with acute asthma?

6. Why is it important to determine what medications the patient might have taken prior to your arrival?

7. In what position should this patient be transported?

BEHAVIORAL EMERGENCIES   25

1. What acute medical disorders commonly mimic behavioral emergencies?

2. Why is it important to determine whether or not an organic disorder exists?

3. What diagnostic maneuvers might you try to eliminate major organic causes?

4. What are the four major categories of behavioral disorders?

5. What are the two types of behavior encountered in the field, and how is each managed

6. What special management techniques must be employed to help the suicidal patient?

7. When are physical restraints indicated and how are they applied?

8. What are the legal considerations involved in handling behavioral emergencies in the prehospital setting?

BURNS 29

1. What vital body functions are impaired when a burn destroys skin layers?

2. What factors determine the severity and treatment of a burn injury?

3. What are the three degrees of burn injury, and how is each identified?

4. How is the extent of burn injury determined in adults? In children?

5. What are the major sources of burn injuries?

6. How are thermal burns treated in the field?

7. How are chemical burns treated in the field?

8. How are electrical burns treated in the field?

9. What are the major contraindications for any burn injury?

10. When should respiratory involvement be suspected, and how is it managed?

11. When should carbon monoxide poisoning be suspected, and how is it managed?

12. What can you do in the field to prevent infection?

13. When should you suspect corneal abrasions, and what should you do about them?

14. Which categories of patients require transport, regardless of the extent of the burn injury?

CARDIAC ARREST 36

1. What are the major causes of cardiac arrest? Respiratory arrest?

2. What arrhythmias usually underly a full cardiac arrest?

3. How is the arrest state confirmed?

4. When should CPR be initiated? When should it not be started?

5. What elements are included in management of the ABCs

6. In addition to controlling ABCs, what general management procedures must also be carried out?

7. When should resuscitative measures be terminated?

8. How is the resuscitation process modified to treat a trauma-induced cardiac arrest?

CEREBROVASCULAR ACCIDENT 40

1. What physiological events cause CVA, and what are some of the precipitating factors?

2. What are the common presenting signs/symptoms of CVA?

3. What is a transient ischemic attack (TIA) and how does it differ from CVA?

4. What is the field management of CVA? Of TIA?

CHEST PAIN (Non-Traumatic) 43

1. What are the two major categories of non-traumatic chest pain?

2. What causes angina pectoris?

3. What are the major sign/symptoms of angina?

4. How is angina treated in the field?

5. What is the physiological basis for acute myocardial infarction (MI)?

6. What is the classic description of MI pain?

7. What other signs/symptoms present with MI?

8. Why are arrhythmias so important in the patient with MI?

9. What clinical finding would lead you to suspect the MI patient had developed cardiogenic shock?

10. What is the field treatment of cardiogenic shock?

11. What is the field treatment of acute MI?

12. What is the physiological basis for dissecting/ruptured aortic aneurysm?

13. What are the signs/symptoms of aneurysm and how is it treated?

14. What is a characteristic description of the pain associated with dissecting aneurysm?

15. What is pericarditis and how will it present in the field?

16. What is the field management of pericarditis?

17. What is pulmonary embolism, and what are the major signs/symptoms?

18. What causes spontaneous pneumothorax, and how does it present?

19. What is pleurisy, and what are the signs/symptoms?

20. What is pneumonia, and what are its major signs/symptoms?

21. What is the field treatment for pulmonary embolism? For spontaneous pneumothorax? For pleurisy? For pneumonia?

CHEST TRAUMA   48

1. What are the three major categories of trauma involving the chest?

2. What is a cardiac contusion; what causes it and what are the presenting signs/symptoms?

3. What is the treatment of cardiac contusion?

4. What is pericardial tamponade; what causes it and what are the presenting signs/symptoms?

5. What is the field treatment of pericardial tamponade?

6. What causes traumatic pneumothorax/hemothorax; what are the resultant signs/symptoms?

7. What is the field treatment for traumatic pneumothorax/hemothorax?

8. How does tension pneumothorax differ from simple pneumothorax?

9. What are the signs/symptoms of tension pneumothorax?

10. What is the field treatment for tension pneumothorax?

11. What is flail chest; what causes it and what are the signs/symptoms confirming it?

12. What is the field treatment of flail chest?

13. What is a sucking chest wound; what causes it and how is it recognized?

14. What is the field treatment of sucking chest wound?

15. What major problems are associated with ruptured ventricle or trauma to the great vessels?

16. How are ruptured ventricle and great vessel trauma recognized?

17. How are ruptured ventricle and great vessel trauma treated?

CHILD ABUSE 53

1. What is child abuse?

2. What criteria are included in the index of suspicion for child abuse?

3. What should be included in your assessment of a child suspected of having been abused?

4. What specific precautions must you take to avoid arousing parental suspicion during your assessment and management of the abused child?

5. How is the abused child managed in the prehospital setting?

6. What are the paramedic's obligations for reporting suspected child abuse?

7. Why is it so critical that the child be transported?

CHRONIC OBSTRUCTIVE PULMONARY DISEASE 56

1. What is COPD; what two disorders are included in this category?

2. What is the pathophysiology of emphysema; what clinical signs/symptoms does it present?

3. What is the pathophysiology of chronic bronchitis; what signs/symptoms does it present?

4. How is oxygen therapy modified for treatment of COPD patients; why?

5. What is the field treatment for acute respiratory distress in a COPD patient?

6. What action is required if the acute COPD patient is not responding to low-flow oxygen?

COLD INJURIES   57

1. What factors influence the severity of a cold injury?

2. What conditions precipitate cold injuries?

3. What are the two major categories of cold injuries?

4. What is the pathophysiology of frostbite?

6. What is the field treatment of frostbite?

7. What procedures are contraindicated in managing frostbite?

8. What is the pathophysiology of systemic hypothermia?

9. What are the signs and symptoms of systemic hypothermia, and what is their order of presentation?

10. What is the field treatment of hypothermia?

11. What is the effect of hypothermia on resuscitation potential?

COMA OF UNKNOWN ORIGIN   61

1. What is coma, and what can cause it?

2. What should be included in your assessment of the unconscious patient?

3. Why should you limit your diagnostic efforts in the field?

4. What two diagnostic maneuvers are justifiable because they identify disorders that are very common and easy to correct?

5. What is the field management of the coma patient?

DIABETES   63

1. What role does insulin play in glucose metabolism?

2. What physiological changes cause the diabetic condition of hypoglycemia (Insulin Shock)?

3. What physiological changes cause the diabetic condition of hyperglycemia (Diabetic Ketoacidosis)?

4. What are the signs/symptoms of Insulin Shock?

5. What are the signs/symptoms of Diabetic Ketoacidosis?

6. What clues from the scene can help you identify an unconscious patient as a diabetic?

7. How would you treat an unconscious diabetic?

8. How would you treat a conscious diabetic who still has an active gag reflex?

9. What procedure should you perform prior to administering any form of glucose?

DIVING ACCIDENTS 68

1. How does the changing atmospheric pressure cause medical problems in scuba divers?

2. What are the two major types of scuba diving accidents?

3. What is the physiologic basis for air embolism among divers?

4. What are the signs and symptoms of air embolism?

5. What specific management procedures are appropriate for a diver who is suffering from air embolism?

6. What is the physiologic basis for decompression sickness?

7. What are the signs and symptoms of decompression sickness?

8. What factors influence the severity of decompression sickness?

9. How is decompression sickness treated in the field?

10. Why is recompression so important to the management of both air embolism and decompression sickness?

11. In what position should victims of diving accidents be transported?

DROWNING 71

1. What are the two major clinical problems associated with near-drowning?

2. What factors affect the severity of the near-drowning patient?

3. What symptoms are commonly associated with near-drowning?

4. How should symptomatic near-drowning patients be managed in the field?

5. How should asymptomatic near-drowning patients be treated?

6. Why is transport so important for all near-drowning victims?

HEAT EXPOSURE 74

1. What are the three primary stages of heat exposure injury?

2. What are the general signs/symptoms associated with all heat exposure injuries?

3. What are heat cramps, and how are they treated?

4. What is heat exhaustion, and how is it treated?

5. What is heat stroke, and how is it treated?

6. What general treatment procedures should be provided all heat injury patients?

HYPERTENSIVE CRISIS 77

1. What are the components of the syndrome known as hypertensive crisis?

2. What are the possible complications of hypertensive crisis?

3. What is included in field treatment of hypertensive crisis?

4. Why is it important to avoid a sudden drop in blood pressure in these patients?

HYPERVENTILATION SYNDROME 79

1. What constitutes the clinical syndrome known as hyperventilation?

2. What other medical conditions can present with hyperventilation as a symptom?

3. Why is it important to differentiate between hyperventilation as a symptom of underlying medical disorder, and a purely emotion-induced hyperventilation syndrome?

4. What should be included in your field assessment of a patient experiencing hyperventilation?

5. What is included in the field treatment of emotion-induced hyperventilation syndrome?

6. If the patient does not readily respond to your initial treatment, what should be your next action?

NEUROLOGICAL TRAUMA 81

1. Why is it important to perform a brief but comprehensive neurological assessment in patients suffering from neurological trauma?

2. What should be included in your field neurological assessment?

3. What are the signs and symptoms of increased intracranial pressure?

4. What should be included in your field treatment of head trauma?

5. What are the signs/symptoms of spinal cord injury?

6. How should spinal cord trauma be managed in the field?

OBSTETRICAL EMERGENCIES 85

1. What criteria would you use to determine whether or not you had time to transport the mother before delivery?

2. How would you prepare the mother for a clean-as-possible field delivery?

3. What steps should you perform to assist the mother in a normal childbirth?

4. What immediate newborn care is required following a normal delivery?

5. How is the placenta delivered, and what should be done if it is not progressing as it should?

6. How would you manage an umbilical cord wrapped around the baby's neck?

7. What is the appropriate field management for a prolapsed cord?

8. How do you alter your assistance if the birth is breech?

9. What should you do to prepare for and manage a multiple birth?

10. How is a normal newborn assessed and managed?

11. How is resuscitation adapted to a newborn?

12. What signs/symptoms are suggestive of post-partum hemorrhage?

13. How is post-partum hemorrhage managed in the field?

14. What clinical signs would suggest to you that a pregnant woman was experiencing toxemia of pregnancy, and how would you treat her?

15. What are the most common causes of vaginal bleeding during pregnancy, and how is it managed?

16. What are common causes of vaginal bleeding in the non-pregnant woman, and what is the appropriate treatment?

OVERDOSE 91

1. What agents are commonly involved in drug overdose?

2. What factors influence severity of the overdose?

3. What should be included in your field management of the overdose patient?

4. What clues from the environment might help you in managing the overdose patient?

5. How is the unconscious overdose patient treated?

6. How does Narcan work in treating overdose patients?

7. How would you treat a conscious overdose patient who has an active gag reflex?

8. How might you modify your treatment processes to manage overdose of hallucinogenic street drugs?

POISONING 95

1. What are the three primary routes of entry of poisonous substances?

2. What are the local effects of poisoning? The systemic effects?

3. What are your primary responsibilities in general management of a poisoned patient?

4. How would you treat a conscious patient who has ingested a caustic substance or a petroleum distillate?

5. How would you treat a conscious patient who has ingested non-caustic substances?

6. What should be included in the treatment of a patient who has ingested narcotics or unknown substances, who is now unconscious or losing consciousness?

7. What should be included in the field management of a patient who ingested substances known to be non-narcotic, and who is now unconscious or losing consciousness?

8. How is organophosphate poisoning recognized?

9. What should be included in the field treatment of organophosphate poisoning?

10. Why is it critical that a patient exposed to organophosphates be transported?

PULMONARY EDEMA 103

1. What is the pathophysiology of pulmonary edema?

2. What common clinical conditions have pulmonary edema as a presenting symptom?

3. What are the characteristic findings associated with pulmonary edema?

4. How does congestive heart failure cause pulmonary edema?

5. What should be included in the field treatment of pulmonary edema?

RADIATION EXPOSURE 105

1. What are likely circumstances in which paramedics would be called to manage a patient exposed to radiation?

2. What factors influence the severity of radiation exposure?

3. What signs/symptoms are associated with radiation exposure?

4. What should be included in the field management of a radiation incident?

5. How does radiation exposure alter your priorities for management of underlying illness/injury?

6. What procedures can you follow to minimize spread of radioactive contaminants?

7. What steps should you take throughout a radiation accident to ensure personal safety and reduce personal exposure?

RAPE AND SEXUAL ASSAULT 109

1. What act(s) constitute rape?

2. What types of people are raped?

3. What are the two major categories of management concerns for the rape victim?

4. What types of physical injury might be involved in a rape?

5. What types of emotional presentation might the patient display?

6. What should be included in the field management of rape?

7. What behaviors/actions should be avoided in the management of a rape victim?

8. What special considerations are required for male rape victims? For geriatric rape victims? For pediatric rape victims?

9. What is the paramedic's role in preserving the victim's legal rights?

SEIZURES 112

1. What is a seizure?

2. What kinds of conditions can cause seizures?

3. What are the major types of seizures, and how is each identified?

4. What are the common phases of a seizure?

5. What should be included in your assessment of seizure activity?

6. What is included in field management of seizure activity?

7. What is status epilepticus, and how is it treated?

SHOCK (Hypovolemic) 116

1. What is the pathophysiology of hypovolemic shock?

2. What kinds of conditions can cause hypovolemic shock?

3. What are the signs/symptoms of hypovolemic shock?

4. What should be included in the field treatment of hypovolemic shock?

SMOKE/GAS INHALATION 118

1. What are the three primary mechanisms by which toxic inhalation produces symptoms?

2. What are the general signs/symptoms associated with toxic inhalation?

3. What general field treatment is indicated for smoke/gas inhalation?

4. What specific signs/symptoms does carbon monoxide poisoning produce?

5. What environmental factors should lead you to suspect CO poisoning?

6. What is included in the field treatment of CO poisoning?

7. What interventions are contraindicated in smoke/gas inhalation?

TRAUMA (Multi-System) 121

1. How does multi-system trauma differ from simpler forms of trauma?

2. What factors should be included in your assessment of the ABCs in a multi-system trauma patient?

3. What elements are included in management of airway, breathing, and circulation in the multi-system trauma patient?

4. Why is prompt transport so important in a multi-system trauma patient?

VENOMOUS LAND ANIMALS 124

1. How do you determine whether or not envenomation occurred during a snakebite?

2. What factors influence severity of injury following snakebite?

3. What are the signs/symptoms associated with envenomation from pit vipers (rattlesnakes, water moccasins, and copperheads)?

4. What signs/symptoms are associated with envenomation from coral snakes?

5. What should be included in your treatment of snakebite injury?

6. What are the two most common poisonous spiders in North America?

7. What signs/symptoms are associated with bites from poisonous spiders?

8. What should be included in your treatment of bites from poisonous spiders?

VENOMOUS WATER ANIMALS 128

1. How do stingray injuries usually occur?

2. What is the character of the injury caused by stingray?

3. What should be done to manage the skin trauma caused by the stingray spine?

4. What types of symptoms might be associated with stingray injury?

5. What can be done to minimize the pain of the stingray injury?

6. What is the general treatment appropriate for stingray injury?

7. How do coelenterates (jellyfish, corals, sea anenomes) cause injury?

8. What are the signs/symptoms of coelenterate envenomation?

9. What should be included in your field treatment of coelenterate injury?

10. What should be done if the patient begins experiencing signs or symptoms of allergic reaction?

SECTION II:
PHARMACOLOGY

CONTENTS

Antibiotics
Anticoagulants
Anticonvulsants
Antidepressants
Antidiarrheal Agents
Antiemetic Agents
Antihistamines
Antihypertensive Agents
Antipsychotic Agents
Antispasmodics
Antituberculosis Agents
Bronchodilators
Cardiac Glycosides
Diuretics
Hormones
Hypoglycemic Agents
Laxatives and Stool Softeners
Sedatives and Hypnotics
Steroids

INTRODUCTION

This section contains individual profiles on a wide range of medications commonly used by paramedics and generally carried on emergency vehicles. Although the specific drugs, dosages, routes and indications may vary in your particular area, we have made an attempt to provide a rapid but complete review of these medications with emphasis on their pre-hospital application. These drug profiles are not intended to teach all there is to know about the pharmacological agents you carry but are intended to supplement and reinforce your present knowledge.

Remember that these medications are potent chemicals that can cause patient deterioration or even death if used improperly. You must have a thorough knowledge of all the medications you carry to avoid errors in administration. The actions, dosages, routes, indications, side effects, and other pertinent information should be committed to memory. Each time you receive a drug order, review your knowledge of the drug to be sure it is being administered properly. Question all orders that you are unsure of, and don't hesitate to question or even refuse an order if you feel it would be detrimental to the patient.

A section has been included on drugs commonly found in the home. This reference is indexed to provide ready information on the indications and actions of drugs which the emergency patient may be taking on a daily basis.

For greater accuracy, pediatric drug dosages are always calculated by the child's weight in kilograms. When calculating pediatric drug dosages, remember that the pediatric dose should never exceed the adult dose range.

The dosages used conform to current standards for Advanced Cardiac Life Support as designated by the American Heart Association. At press time, the most current AHA publication was "Textbook of Advanced Cardiac Life Support", K. McIntyre and A. J. Lewis, editors, AHA, Dallas, TX, 1981. Due to rapid advances and frequent changes in emergency medical care, it is recommended that the dosages and other pertinent information in this section be updated on a regular basis.

---

*This listing does not purport to be an endorsement by the authors of any of the drugs mentioned herein.

AMINOPHYLLINE

(Theophylline ethelenediamine)

CLASS: bronchodilator

INDICATIONS:
- asthma, status asthmaticus
- pulmonary edema with associated wheezing
- C.O.P.D.

ACTION:
- relaxes smooth muscles
  - bronchodilator
  - vasodilator
  - mild diuretic
- stimulates cardiovascular system
- stimulates central nervous system
- enhances respiratory drive

DOSAGE/ ROUTE:
- 3–6 mg/kg in at least 20 ml D5W IV drip via Volutrol over a minimum of 20 minutes
- usual range 250–500mg

SIDE EFFECTS:
- PVC's, PAC's and tachycardias
- hypotension (transient)
- seizure activity
- nausea and/or vomiting

CONTRA- INDICATIONS:
- hypotension

SPECIAL INFORMATION:
- If patient is taking any theophylline preparation dosage should be reduced
- rapid infusion may cause seizure activity, cardiac irritability and/or arrest
- hypoxic patients are more prone to develop side effects
- check lung sounds for effectiveness of the drug
- monitor EKG
- check blood pressure frequently

PEDIATRIC DOSAGE:
- Epinephrine is drug of choice for asthma
- same as adult dosage
- use with caution in children under age 12

AMMONIA AMPULES

(Ammonia Inhalant, Aromatic Spirits of Ammonia)

CLASS: respiratory stimulant

INDICATIONS:
- syncope
- to determine level of consciousness

ACTION:
- elicits a response in a conscious patient by irritating mucous membranes of upper respiratory tract
- stimulates vasomotor center of the medulla causing an increase in blood pressure

DOSAGE/ ROUTE:
- 2–3 inhalations; break ampule and hold close to patient's nostrils

SIDE EFFECTS:
- none

CONTRA-INDICATIONS:
- none

SPECIAL INFORMATION:
- Use with caution in patients with COPD or asthma—may cause bronchospasms.
- Be sure patient has inhaled sufficient vapor to elicit a response.

PEDIATRIC DOSAGE: same as adult

ARAMINE

(Metaraminol Bitartrate)

CLASS: vasopressor

INDICATIONS:
- acute hypotension

ACTION:
- constricts blood vessels
- increases myocardial contractility

**DOSAGE/
ROUTE:**
- 100 mg in 250 ml 5% D/W (0.4 mg/ml); titrate to blood pressure and tissue perfusion

**SIDE
EFFECTS:**
- hypertension
- tachycardia
- ventricular irritability
- reflex bradycardia
- decreased renal, cerebral, and coronary blood flow

**CONTRA-
INDICATIONS:**
- hypovolemia (should not be given until fluid replacement is attempted)

**SPECIAL
INFORMATION:**
- start IV drip at low infusion rate and increase gradually to prevent hypertension and cardiac arrest
- because of its profound effects on the heart, kidneys and periphery use with caution in cardiac and diabetic patients
- if infiltration occurs discontinue IV drip, circle area of infiltration, and report to hospital–tissue necrosis is rare possibility
- less potent and longer lasting than Levophed

**PEDIATRIC
DOSAGE:**
- 50–100 mg in 250 ml 5% D/W; start at 0.4 mg/kg, titrate to blood pressure

ATROPINE

(Atropine Sulfate)

CLASS: anticholinergic

INDICATIONS:
- sinus bradycardia with severe hypotension or frequent PVCs
- sinus bradycardia without hypotension or PVCs if rate is less than 50 beats/min
- high degree AV block at nodal level
- ventricular asystole
- organophosphate poisoning

ACTION:
- competes with acetycholine for receptor sites at

the synapse, thus blocking the parasympathetic response
- increases electrical conduction through the heart
- inhibits secretion

DOSAGE/ ROUTE:
- cardiac arrhythmias:
  0.5 mg IV push; repeat as needed every 5 minutes up to a maximum of 2 mg; a 1 mg. bolus can be given initially in asystole
- organophosphate poisoning:
  2 mg IV push or IM, may repeat as needed

SIDE EFFECTS:
- tachycardia
- dries mucous membranes
- dilates pupils
- toxicity: flushed skin; restlessness; decreased level of consciousness; irritability; hallucinations

CONTRA- INDICATIONS:
- none

SPECIAL INFORMATION:
- use with caution in patients with MI (can extend infarct) or glaucoma (increases intraocular pressure)
- monitor EKG closely
- may suppress PVC's seen in a sinus bradycardia by overriding the irritable ectopic focus
- atropine will not reverse the muscle weakness associated with organophosphate poisoning—the drug PAM (protopam) is used for this purpose

PEDIATRIC DOSAGE:
- cardiac arrhythmias:
  0.01–0.03 mg/kg IV push, may repeat
- organophosphate poisoning:
  0.05 mg/kg IV push or IM; may repeat

BENADRYL

(Diphenhydramine Hydrochloride)

CLASS: antihistamine

INDICATIONS:
- allergic reactions/anaphylaxis (after administration of epinephrine)
- idiosyncratic reaction to thorazine, compazine and other related drugs (extrapyramidal reaction)

ACTION:
- binds to histamine receptor sites to prevent further allergic reaction
- causes sedation

DOSAGE/ ROUTE:
- 25–50 mg slow IV push or deep IM

SIDE EFFECTS:
- drowsiness, syncope
- hypotension
- thickened mucous secretions
- toxicity: seizures, coma and death

CONTRA- INDICATIONS:
- asthma attack
- infants under 20 pounds

SPECIAL INFORMATION:
- cumulative depressant effects occur in presence of alcohol and/or other sedatives

PEDIATRIC DOSAGE:
2 mg/kg slow IV push or deep IM

BRETYLIUM

(Bretylium tosylate, Bretylol)

CLASS: antiarrhythmic

INDICATIONS:
- ventricular fibrillation (facilitates termination of VF by DC countershock)
- ventricular tachycardia
- only indicated if other forms of therapy have failed to control the arrhythmia

ACTION:
- increases ventricular fibrillation threshhold
- decreases re-entry phenomenon

DOSAGE/ ROUTE:
Ventricular Fibrillation
- rapid IV Push: 5 mg/kg (500 mg average dose);

defibrillate; then give 10 mg/kg if needed; may repeat at 15–30 min intervals to a maximum of 30 mg/kg
- IV Drip: 1–2 mg/min after loading dose

Ventricular Tachycardia
500 mg in 50 ml; inject 5–10 mg/kg IV push over 8–10 min; follow by IV drip of 1–2 mg/min

SIDE EFFECTS:
- postural hypotension following conversion
- nausea/vomiting after rapid injection in a conscious patient

CONTRA-INDICATIONS:
- children
- digitalis toxicity

SPECIAL INFORMATION:
- onset of action is within minutes in VF; can be delayed 20 min or more in VT
- does not alter conduction velocity or depress cardiac contractility
- once patient converts, monitor blood pressure closely

PEDIATRIC DOSAGE:
safety and efficacy of use has not been established

CALCIUM

($CaCl_2$, Calcium Chloride 10%)

CLASS:
electrolyte

INDICATIONS:
- electromechanical dissociation
- asystole after the administration of sodium bicarbonate and epinephrine

ACTION:
- improves myocardial contractility
- may enhance ventricular automaticity

DOSAGE/ ROUTE:
- 5–7 mg/kg IV push; may repeat every 10 min if necessary (usual dosage 250–500 mg)

SIDE EFFECTS:
- none expected with normal use

CONTRA-INDICATIONS:	• none

SPECIAL INFORMATION:	• use with caution in patients taking digitalis preparations • precipitates if mixed with $NaHCO_3$ • potent local irritant

PEDIATRIC DOSAGE:	• 0.3 ml/kg (of 10% solution) IV push

DECADRON

(Dexamethazone, Dezone, Hexadrol Phosphate)

CLASS:	• synthetic adrenocortical steroid • anti-inflammatory agent

INDICATIONS:	• acute cerebral edema • shock

ACTION:	exact mechanism is unclear

DOSAGE/ ROUTE:	10–20 mg IV push

SIDE EFFECTS:	• anaphylaxis • hypertension • thromboembolism • hyperglycemia • peptic ulcer perforation and hemorrhage

CONTRA-INDICATIONS:	diabetes, pregnancy, renal insufficiency, thrombolic tendencies, myasthenia gravis, acute psychosis

SPECIAL INFORMATION:	• onset for acute cerebral edema is 4–6 hours • action is inhibited by phenytoin • incompatible with other drugs • sensitive to temperature extremes

PEDIATRIC DOSAGE:	0.08–0.3 mg/kg over a 24-hour period

DEXTROSE, 5% IN WATER

(5% DW, D5W, 5DW)

CLASS:	crystalloid

INDICATIONS:
- mainly used to keep open a vein
- life-line for administration of medications
- for dilution of IV drip drugs

ACTION:
- provides glucose solution for parenteral therapy

DOSAGE/ ROUTE:
- IV drip, regulated according to patient condition

SIDE EFFECTS:
- none expected with normal use

CONTRA- INDICATIONS:
- none

SPECIAL INFORMATION:
- content: 50 gm dextrose/liter (170 calories/liter)
- use with caution in head injuries
- use fluids conservatively in patients with pulmo-nary congestion

PEDIATRIC DOSAGE:
- IV drip via Volutrol; regulated according to pa-tient condition

DEXTROSE, 50%

(D50W, 50% Glucose)

CLASS:	carbohydrate

INDICATIONS:
- unconscious diabetic patient
- diagnostic tool in coma, CVA, seizures or behav-ioral disorders

ACTION:
- provides free sugar for quick absorption into blood stream

**DOSAGE/
ROUTE:**
- 25 gm IV push

**SIDE
EFFECTS:**
- none expected with normal use

**CONTRA-
INDICATIONS:**
- none

**SPECIAL
INFORMATION:**
- always draw blood sugar prior to administration
- tissue necrosis occurs with infiltration; make sure injection is intravenous; aspirate before and during injection
- one bolus of 50% dextrose will not adversely effect the hyperglycemic patient

**PEDIATRIC
DOSAGE:**
- 1 ml/kg slow IV push

DIGOXIN

("Dig", Lanoxin)

CLASS: cardiotonic

INDICATIONS:
- uncompensated supraventricular tachycardias
- congestive heart failure

ACTION:
- improves stroke volume
- increases cardiac output
- increases strength of myocardial contraction
- slows conduction at the SA and AV nodes
- lowers myocardial oxygen consumption

**DOSAGE/
ROUTE:**
- 0.5–0.75 mg/45 kg (100 lbs), IV push

**SIDE
EFFECTS:**
- bradycardias
- AV blocks
- toxicity: GI disturbances, visual disturbances, arrhythmias (tachycardia, ventricular bigeminy, PAT with block, sinus arrest)

CONTRA-INDICATIONS:	• none

SPECIAL INFORMATION:
- use caution when administering Calcium Chloride or cardioverting a patient who has received a digitalis preparation
- in patients with supraventricular tachycardias rule out dig-toxicity before treatment

PEDIATRIC DOSAGE:
- Should not be given to children in the field

DOPAMINE

(Dopamine Hydrochloride, Intropin)

CLASS: natural catecholamine (both alpha and beta properties)

INDICATIONS: Shock
- cardiogenic (drug of choice)
- low resistance (septic, anaphylactic)
- hypovolemic (after sufficient volume replacement)

ACTION:
- increases cardiac output by increasing contractility and stroke volume, thereby increasing blood pressure
- selectively dilates blood vessels supplying the brain, kidneys, heart and gastrointestinal tract
- may increase heart rate slightly
- causes significant peripheral vasoconstriction only in very large doses

DOSAGE/ ROUTE: 200 mg in 500 ml 5% D/W (400 mcg/ml IV drip; begin with 2–5 mcg/kg/min; titrate to blood pressure

SIDE EFFECTS:
- ventricular irritability
- hypertension and extreme vasoconstriction can occur with high infusion rates
- hypotension can occur with low infusion rates

**CONTRA-
INDICATIONS:**
- none

**SPECIAL
INFORMATION:**
- titrate to blood pressure and patient response
- tissue necrosis may occur with infiltration, discontinue IV drip, circle area of infiltration and inform hospital
- effects of the drug cease approximately 10 minutes after drip is stopped

**PEDIATRIC
DOSAGE:**
2–10 mcg/kg/min IV drip

EPINEPHRINE

(Adrenalin, "Epi")

CLASS:
natural catecholamine (both alpha and beta properties)

INDICATIONS:
- severe cardiac arrhythmias (asystole, idioventricular rhythm, or ventricular fibrillation)
- asthma attacks
- allergic reaction/anaphylaxis

ACTION:
- increases heart rate, contractility, AV conduction, and myocardial irritability
- produces bronchodilatation
- produces peripheral vasoconstriction

**DOSAGE/
ROUTE:**
- cardiac arrhythmias: 0.5–1 mg 1:10,000 IV push, via ET tube, or IC
- asthma attack: 0.3 mg 1:1,000 SC; may repeat 3 times at 5 minute intervals
- allergic reaction/anaphylaxis: 0.3 mg 1:1,000 SC; may repeat 3 times at 5 minute intervals, *or* if reaction is severe, 0.1–0.5 mg 1:10,000 IV push; may repeat in 10 minutes (not to exceed 0.5 mg in 10 minutes)

**SIDE
EFFECTS:**
- supraventricular tachycardia
- ventricular irritability

CONTRA-INDICATIONS: none

SPECIAL INFORMATION:
- monitor EKG, vital signs, and lung sounds to assess effectiveness
- use with caution in patients with angina and/or hypertension
- may aggravate pre-existing tachycardia
- Aminophylline is drug of choice for asthmatics older than 35 who do not usually take epinephrine
- can induce early labor if given to a pregnant patient

PEDIATRIC DOSAGE:
- cardiac arrhythmias: 0.01 ml/kg 1:10,000 IV push, via ET tube, or IC
- asthma attack: 0.01 ml/kg (1:1,000) SC; may repeat times 3 at 20 minute intervals to a maximum of 0.3 mg
- allergic reaction/anaphylaxis: 0.01 ml/kg (1:1,000) SC; may repeat times 3 at 20 minute intervals to a maximum of 0.3 mg; *or* if reaction is severe, 0.01 mg/kg (1:10,000) IV push; may repeat in 10 minutes (not to exceed 0.5 mg in 10 minutes)

GLUCAGON

(Glucagon Hydrochloride)

CLASS: polypeptide

INDICATIONS: known diabetic who is unconscious, and in whom an IV cannot be established

ACTION: increases blood glucose by converting liver glycogen to glucose

DOSAGE/ ROUTE: 0.5–1 unit IM or SC

SIDE EFFECTS: nausea, vomiting

CONTRA-INDICATIONS:	none for field use

SPECIAL INFORMATION:

- 50% dextrose is drug of choice if IV can be established
- draw blood sugar prior to administration of glucagon; label with patient's name, date, and "pre-glucagon"
- onset of action is 5–20 minutes
- store at room temperature; once reconstituted, must be refrigerated

PEDIATRIC DOSAGE: 50 mcg/kilogram

GLUCOLA

(Carbonated Carbohydrate Solution, Glucose Solution)

CLASS: carbohydrate

INDICATIONS:
- hypoglycemia in an alert patient

ACTION:
- provides free sugar for quick absorption into the blood stream

DOSAGE/ROUTE:
- 75–100 gm orally

SIDE EFFECTS:
- none expected with normal use

CONTRA-INDICATIONS:
- absence of gag reflex

SPECIAL INFORMATION:
- always draw blood sugar prior to administration
- check for presence of gag reflex prior to administration

PEDIATRIC DOSAGE:
- 10–100 gm P.O. based upon weight

INDERAL

(Propranolol)

CLASS: beta blocker

INDICATIONS:
- uncompensated supraventricular tachycardias (after Valsalva's maneuver and/or carotid sinus massage)

ACTION:
- decreases heart rate
- decreases AV conduction
- decreases myocardial contractility
- decreases myocardial oxygen consumption
- suppresses supraventricular and ventricular ectopics
- increases airway resistance

DOSAGE/ ROUTE:
- up to 1 mg slow IV push every 5 minutes, for a total of no more than 5 mg

SIDE EFFECTS:
- bradycardias
- may precipitate congestive heart failure due to decrease in contractility
- transient hypotension

CONTRA- INDICATIONS:
- asthma
- pulmonary edema

SPECIAL INFORMATION:
- use with caution in pregancy and patients on anti-hypertensive or diuretic drugs
- monitor patient closely while administering and watch for arrhythmias

PEDIATRIC DOSAGE: not used in children

IPECAC

(Syrup of Ipecac)

CLASS: emetic

INDICATIONS:
- overdose in an *alert* patient

ACTION:
- irritates lining of stomach
- stimulates vomiting center in the medulla

DOSAGE/ ROUTE:
- 30 ml orally, followed by 8–16 ounces of clear fluid, may repeat in 30 minutes

SIDE EFFECTS:
- none expected with normal use

CONTRA- INDICATIONS:
- ingestion of petroleum distillate
- ingestion of acidic substance
- ingestion of alkaline substance
- absence of gag reflex

SPECIAL INFORMATION:
- check for presence of gag reflex prior to administration
- watch level of consciousness and airway after administration until emesis occurs (onset 20–30 minutes)

PEDIATRIC DOSAGE:
- 15 ml followed by 4–8 ounces of clear fluid

ISUPREL

(Isoproterenol Hydrochloride)

CLASS: synthetic catecholamine (pure beta)

INDICATIONS:
- cardiac 1:5000
  - severe bradycardias
  - AV blocks refractory to atropine
  - idioventricular rhythms
- respiratory 1:400
  - asthma

ACTION:
- increases heart rate
- increases contractility
- speeds SA, AV and ventricular conduction
- increases myocardial oxygen consumption

- produces bronchodilatation
- produces peripheral vasodilatation

**DOSAGE/
ROUTE:**

- cardiac 1:5000
  1 mg in 500 ml 5% D/W IV drip (2 mcg/ml); run
  at 2–20 mcg/min, titrated to pulse
- respiratory inhaler 1:400
  1–2 deep inhalations. Have patient hold inhalation
  for a few seconds before exhaling. May repeat
  once after 5 minutes

**SIDE
EFFECTS:**

- tachycardias
- ventricular irritability
- transient hypotension

**CONTRA-
INDICATIONS:**

- in asthma: preexisting tachyarrhythmias from
  overuse of bronchodilators

**SPECIAL
INFORMATION:**

- use with caution in patients with acute MI
- monitor EKG to determine effectiveness of drug
- check pulse and blood pressure frequently
- when using inhaler, check lung sounds before and
  after administration to determine effectiveness of
  drug
- if Isuprel inhaler does not break asthma attack try
  epinephrine and/or Aminophylline
- report to hospital any use of antiasthmatic drugs
  prior to your arrival (patients frequently overuse
  their inhaler and may develop paradoxical bronchoconstriction)
- Isuprel has a cumulative effect when used with
  epinephrine

**PEDIATRIC
DOSAGE:**

- cardiac: start at 0.1 mcg/kg/min IV drip; titrate to
  blood pressure
- respiratory: same as adult dosage

LASIX

(Furosemide)

CLASS: diuretic

INDICATIONS:
- acute pulmonary edema

ACTION:
- stimulates the kidneys to excrete water, sodium chloride, and potassium which leads to a decreased circulating blood volume
- produces vasodilatation

DOSAGE/ ROUTE:
- 0.5 mg/kg (usual dose 40 mg) slow IV push; may give up to 2 mg/kg if indicated

SIDE EFFECTS:
- transient hypotension

CONTRA- INDICATIONS:
- pregnancy

SPECIAL INFORMATION:
- very potent with rapid onset—5–10 minutes
- generally safe acutely, but prolonged use or large doses can lead to potassium loss with dehydration, hypotension, and cardiac arrhythmias
- if patient is on diuretics, may need a larger dose to reach the desired effect
- check lung sounds before and after administration to determine effectiveness of drug
- patients with known sulfonamide sensitivity may develop an allergic reaction to lasix

PEDIATRIC DOSAGE:
1 mg/kg/dose IV push over 1–4 minutes

LEVOPHED

(Levarterenol Bitartrate, Norepinephrine)

CLASS:
- natural catecholamine (mostly alpha)
- vasopressor

INDICATIONS:
- shock

ACTION:
- potent vasoconstrictor which increases blood pressure by direct effect on peripheral blood vessels

- dilates coronary arteries
- increases myocardial contractility

DOSAGE/ ROUTE: 8 mg in 500 ml 5% D/W or NS (16 mcg/ml) IV drip; start at 2–3 ml/min and titrate to maintain a low-normal blood pressure

SIDE EFFECTS:
- severe hypertension
- bradycardia

CONTRA-INDICATIONS:
- hypovolemia until fluid replacement is attempted

SPECIAL INFORMATION:
- tissue necrosis will occur with infiltration; discontinue IV drip and circle area of infiltration
- increased blood pressure may stimulate baroreceptors, causing a reflex bradycardia
- monitor perfusion parameters—quality of pulses, skin color, temperature, and level of consciousness

PEDIATRIC DOSAGE: start at 0.1 mcg/kg/min IV drip; titrate to blood pressure

LIDOCAINE

(Lidocaine Hydrochloride, 2% Xylocaine)

CLASS: antiarrhythmic

INDICATIONS:
- ventricular irritability (including recurrent or refractory ventricular fibrillation)
- prophylaxis against ventricular fibrillation (in the presence of chest pain)

ACTION: decreases ventricular automaticity

DOSAGE/ ROUTE: *Ventricular Irritability*
- Initial bolus of 1 mg/kg slow IV push, followed immediately by an IV drip of 1–2 Gm in 250–500 ml 5% D/W and run at 2–4 mg/min.

- An additional bolus of 0.5 mg/kg can be given in 10 min if necessary. Each time an additional bolus injection is required, the IV drip rate should be increased by 1 mg/min, up to a maximum of 4 mg/min.
- If an IV drip is not possible or practical, a therapeutic blood level should be maintained with repeated bolus injections.
- The total maximum dosage is 4 mg/kg/hr.

Prophylaxis Against Ventricular Fibrillation
- Initial loading dose of 200 mg, which can be injected as 100 mg over a two-minute period at ten-minute intervals, or as four 50 mg injections at five-minute intervals.
- Simultaneously start an IV drip of 1–2 Gm in 250–500 mg 5% D/W and run at 2–3 mg/min.
- If ventricular irritability persists, give another bolus of 50–100 mg over a 1–2 minute period and increase infusion rate.

SIDE EFFECTS:
toxicity:
Early: anxiety, euphoria, combativeness, nausea, twitchings, numbness
Late: convulsions, decreased blood pressure, coma, widening of QRS complex, prolonged PRI

CONTRA-INDICATIONS:
- idioventricular or escape rhythms
- contraindications for prophylactic use:
  impaired liver function (e.g., CHF, jaundice)
  impaired perfusion (e.g., hypotension, old age)

SPECIAL INFORMATION:
- Use caution in patients with documented conduction system disorders.
- Use one half of the prescribed dosage in the presence of shock or pulmonary edema.
- Acts within 2 minutes and lasts approximately 10–20 minutes from time bolus is given.
- In a bradycardia with PVCs, give atropine before Lidocaine.
- Monitor frequency of ventricular irritability to determine effectiveness of drug.
- Decrease drip rate at first indication of toxicity.

PEDIATRIC DOSAGE:	IV Bolus: 1 mg/kg/dose IV Drip: 30 mcg/kg/min

MANNITOL

(Osmitrol)

CLASS:	osmotic diuretic
INDICATIONS:	• head injury with signs of increased intracranial pressure
ACTION:	• draws fluid from brain cells and intracellular spaces • produces diuresis
DOSAGE/ ROUTE:	• 200 mg/kg IV drip over 3–5 minutes
SIDE EFFECTS:	• dehydration
CONTRA- INDICATIONS:	• renal failure • congestive heart failure
SPECIAL INFORMATION:	• *do not* use if crystals are seen in the solution • use inline filter for administration • monitor vital and neurologic signs closely • use with caution in hypovolemia and pregnancy
PEDIATRIC DOSAGE:	• 200 mg/kg IV over 3–5 min

METAPREL

(Metaproterenol, Alupent, Metaprel Metered Aerosol)

CLASS:	bronchodilator (Beta-2 stimulant)
INDICATIONS:	• asthma • chronic obstructive pulmonary disease

172

ACTION:
- relaxes smooth muscles of the bronchial tree
- stimulates the heart only minimally

**DOSAGE/
ROUTE:**
- 1–2 deep inhalations, may repeat once after 5 minutes
- have patient hold inhalation for a few seconds before exhaling

**SIDE
EFFECTS:**
- tachycardia
- palpitations
- PVC's

**CONTRA-
INDICATIONS:**
- pre-existing tachyarrhythmias from overuse of bronchodilators

**SPECIAL
INFORMATION:**
- check lung sounds before and after administration to determine effectiveness of drug
- report to hospital any use of antiasthmatic drugs prior to your arrival (patients frequently overuse their inhaler and may develop paradoxical bronchoconstriction)
- monitor EKG
- use with caution in pregnancy

**PEDIATRIC
DOSAGE:**
- not recommended for children under 12 yrs of age

MORPHINE

(MS, MSO4, Morphine Sulfate)

CLASS:
- narcotic/analgesic
- CNS depressant

INDICATIONS:
- myocardial infarction
- pulmonary edema
- burns
- isolated injuries

ACTION:
- decreases pain perception and anxiety
- relaxes respiratory effort
- produces peripheral vasodilatation, thereby decreasing blood return to the heart

● increases vagal tone

**DOSAGE/
ROUTE:**

Slow IV Push	IM
2–5 mg may repeat every 5–30 min; titrate to effect	5–15 mg based on patient's weight

**SIDE
EFFECTS:**
● respiratory depression and/or arrest
● decreased level of consciousness
● transient hypotension
● bradycardia
● nausea/vomiting

**CONTRA-
INDICATIONS:**
● hypotension
● head injury
● abdominal pain
● multiple trauma
● chronic lung disease
● compromised respirations

**SPECIAL
INFORMATION:**
● monitor vital signs closely
● Narcan will reverse overdose effects

**PEDIATRIC
DOSAGE:**
● 0.1–0.2 mg/kg IV push over 3–5 minutes; titrate to effect

NARCAN

(Naloxone)

CLASS: narcotic antagonist

INDICATIONS:
● symptomatic narcotic overdose
● diagnostic tool in coma of unknown origin

ACTION:
● reverses respiratory depression as well as other effects of narcotic overdose by occupying opiate receptor sites

**DOSAGE/
ROUTE:**
- 0.4–0.8 mg IV push or IM; may repeat as many as 10–15 times

**SIDE
EFFECTS:**
- none expected with normal use

**CONTRA-
INDICATIONS:**
- none

**SPECIAL
INFORMATION:**
- quick onset of action (30 seconds to 2 minutes)
- onset of action for IM dose is within 2 minutes
- initial response may be temporary; watch for a relapse as long as the narcotic is still in the patient's system
- Narcan can precipitate withdrawal syndrome and/or combative behavior
- do not insert esophageal airway prior to administration of Narcan
- effective against natural and synthetic narcotics, including:

Codeine	Lomotil
Darvon	Methadone
Demerol	Morphine
Dilaudid	Paregoric
Heroin	Percodan

**PEDIATRIC
DOSAGE:**
0.01 mg/kg/dose IV push or IM; may repeat as necessary

NITROGLYCERINE

(NTG, TNT, Nitro)

CLASS: vasodilator

INDICATIONS:
- angina pectoris

ACTION:
- produces systemic vasodilation thereby causing decreased right heart return
- decreases myocardial workload
- decreases myocardial oxygen consumption

**DOSAGE/
ROUTE:**
- 0.4 mg (1/150 gr) sublingual, may repeat at 3–5 min intervals as necessary, up to a total of 3 tablets

**SIDE
EFFECTS:**
- transient hypotension (can be profound)
- temporary pulsating headache
- facial flushing

**CONTRA-
INDICATIONS:**
- hypotension
- children under 12 years of age

**SPECIAL
INFORMATION:**
- place patient in supine position before administering drug
- always check blood pressure before and after administration
- store in a dark place to maintain potency
- replace 30 days after opening bottle
- effective in 1–2 min; effects last up to 30 minutes

**PEDIATRIC
DOSAGE:**
not used in children

NORMAL SALINE

(NS, Saline, 0.9% Sodium Chloride, Physiologic Saline, NaCl)

CLASS:
crystalloid

INDICATIONS:
- hypovolemia
- prophylactically in situations where hypovolemia is anticipated
- dehydration
- eye irrigant

ACTION:
- increases circulating volume by remaining in the vascular system

**DOSAGE/
ROUTE:**
- IV drip, regulated according to patient condition

**SIDE
EFFECTS:**
- none expected with normal use

CONTRA-INDICATIONS:
- pulmonary edema

SPECIAL INFORMATION:
- content: 154 mEq Na/liter
  154 mEq Cl/liter
- use fluids conservatively in patients with suspected head injuries

PEDIATRIC DOSAGE:
- IV drip, via Volutrol, regulated according to body weight and patient condition

PITOCIN

(Oxytocin, "Pit")

CLASS: oxytocic

INDICATIONS:
- postpartum hemorrhage

ACTION:
- constricts uterine musculature, thereby compressing uterine blood vessels and reducing blood flow

DOSAGE/ ROUTE:

IM	IV Drip
3–10 units	10–20 units in 1000 ml Ringer's Lactate; titrate to severity of hemorrhage and uterine response

SIDE EFFECTS: uterine cramping

CONTRA-INDICATIONS:
- administration prior to delivery of both the infant and placenta

SPECIAL INFORMATION:
- if administered prior to delivery of infant and placenta, uterus may rupture with subsequent maternal and infant death

- use with extreme caution in patients with previous Cesarean section or uterine surgery
- uterine effect occurs within 1 minute and lasts up to 30 minutes after the infusion is discontinued
- to be used in conjunction with other methods of postpartum hemorrhage control such as fluid replacement, uterine massage, baby to breast, shock position and anti-shock trousers

PEDIATRIC DOSAGE: not established

RINGER'S LACTATE

(Lactated Ringer's Solution, R/L, L/R)

CLASS: crystalloid

INDICATIONS:
- hypovolemia
- prophylactically in situations where hypovolemia is anticipated
- dehydration

ACTION:
- increases circulating volume by remaining in the vascular system

DOSAGE/ ROUTE:
- IV drip, regulated according to patient condition

SIDE EFFECTS:
- none expected with normal use

CONTRA- INDICATIONS:
- pulmonary edema

SPECIAL INFORMATION:
- content per liter:
  - 130 mEq Na
  - 109 mEq Cl
  - 4 mEq K
  - 3 mEq Ca
  - 28 mEq lactate
- use fluids conservatively in patients with suspected head injuries

PEDIATRIC DOSAGE:
- IV drip, via Volutrol, regulated according to body weight and patient condition

SODIUM BICARBONATE

("Bicarb", NaHCO₃)

CLASS: alkalotic agent

INDICATIONS:
- cardiopulmonary arrest

ACTION:
- reduces acidosis by direct release of base radicals into the blood stream

DOSAGE/ ROUTE:
- 1 mEq/kg IV push initially, and no more than half this dose every 10 minutes of continued arrest

SIDE EFFECTS:
- none expected with normal use

CONTRA-INDICATIONS:
- none

SPECIAL INFORMATION:
- precipitates if mixed with calcium chloride; flush tubing between administration of drugs
- alkalosis occurs if given too frequently or in a patient being well ventilated

PEDIATRIC DOSAGE: 1–2 mEq/kg/dose

VALIUM

(Diazepam)

CLASS:
- anticonvulsant
- sedative

INDICATIONS:
- sustained and/or recurrent grand mal seizures
- precardioversion to reduce anxiety and decrease recall

- acute behavioral disorders

ACTION:
- decreases cerebral irritability
- produces sedation
- relaxes skeletal muscles

DOSAGE/ ROUTE:
- IV Push: 2.5–20 mg in 2.5 mg increments, over 1 minute, titrated to effect
- IM: 5–10 mg

SIDE EFFECTS:
- respiratory depression or arrest
- drowsiness
- vertigo
- transient hypotension

CONTRA-INDICATIONS:
- neonates less than 30 days old
- acute narrow angle glaucoma

SPECIAL INFORMATION:
- causes respiratory arrest if given too fast or too much
- use with caution in shock states and pregnant women
- precipitates when mixed or diluted with another drug or IV solution; when giving IV push, inject as close to needle as possible to prevent precipitation in tubing
- is very painful during administration
- has a cumulative effect with alcohol and sedatives

PEDIATRIC DOSAGE:
- 0.25 mg/kg slow IV push over a 3-minute period; may repeat once after 15–30 minutes; don't use in neonates less than 30 days old.

SELF-ASSESSMENT
QUESTIONS

AMINOPHYLLINE 153

1. What are the indications for field use of Aminophylline?

2. What are the main actions of Aminophylline?

3. What is the dose and route of administration of Aminophylline?

4. What are the side effects of Aminophylline?

5. When is Aminophylline contraindicated?

6. What arrhythmias are commonly seen with the administration of Aminophylline?

7. How is the effectiveness of Aminophylline determined?

8. What is the drug of choice in a child who is having an asthma attack?

9. What is the pediatric dosage of Aminophylline?

AMMONIA AMPULES 154

1. When is it appropriate to use Ammonia Ampules?

2. How does Ammonia work?

3. In which patients should Ammonia Ampules be used with caution?

4. How is an Ammonia Ampule administered?

5. Is the dosage of Ammonia altered if the patient is a child?

ARAMINE 154–155

1. When is Aramine indicated?

2. How does Aramine work?

3. What is the dosage and route of Aramine?

4. What side effects can occur if Aramine is given too rapidly?

5. When is Aramine contraindicated?

6. Which arrhythmias can be caused by the administration of Aramine?

7. Why must the Aramine flow rate be increased *gradually?*

8. What is the pediatric dose of Aramine?

ATROPINE   155–156

1. When is Atropine indicated?

2. What are the actions of Atropine?

3. What is the dosage and route of Atropine for cardiac arrhythmias? For organophosphate poisoning?

4. What are the signs and symptoms of Atropine toxicity?

5. Why should Atropine be used with caution in glaucoma patients? In MI patients?

6. How is Atropine used to treat PVCs in a bradycardia?

7. What is the pediatric dose of Atropine for cardiac arrhythmias? For organophosphate poisoning?

BENADRYL   156–157

1. What are the field indications for Benadryl?

2. How does Benadryl work against anaphylaxis?

3. Benadryl is used as an antidote against what group of drugs?

4. What are the dosage and routes of Benadryl?

5. What are the major side effects of Benadryl?

6. What are the signs of Benadryl toxicity?

7. Why is Benadryl contraindicated in an asthma attack?

8. Benadryl has a cumulative effect with what group of drugs?

9. What is the pediatric dose of Benadryl?

BRETYLIUM   157–158

1. What are the primary uses for Bretylium?

2. What is the action of Bretylium?

3. At what stage of treatment is it appropriate to use Bretylium?

4. What is the dosage and route of Bretylium for ventricular fibrillation? For ventricular tachycardia?

5. What are the side effects of Bretylium?

6. When is Bretylium contraindicated?

7. What is the pediatric dose of Bretylium?

CALCIUM CHLORIDE   158–159

1. When is Calcium indicated?

2. What are the actions of Calcium?

3. What is the dose and routes of Calcium?

4. Why is Calcium given in electromechanical dissociation?

5. Why should Calcium be administered slowly when given IV push?

6. What complication can occur if Calcium is administered with Sodium Bicarbonate?

7. Calcium should be used with caution in patients on which medication?

8. What is the pediatric dose of Calcium?

DECADRON   159

1. What are the primary emergency uses of Decadron?

2. What is the dosage and route of Decadron?

3. What are the contraindications to use of Decadron?

4. What are some of the side effects of Decadron?

5. Why must Decadron be maintained at an even temperature?

6. What is Decadron's onset of action for acute cerebral edema?

7. What drug inhibits the action of Decadron?

8. What is the pediatric dose of Decadron?

DEXTROSE (5%) IN WATER   160

1. What class of IV solution is 5% D/W?

2. When would 5% D/W be indicated rather than another IV solution?

3. When should 5% D/W be used with caution?

DEXTROSE (50%)   160–161

1. When is 50% Dextrose indicated?

2. What is the action of 50% Dextrose?

3. What is the usual dose and route of 50% Dextrose?

4. What complication can occur if 50% Dextrose infiltrates? How can this complication be avoided?

5. What procedure should precede the administration of any glucose solution? Why?

6. What is the pediatric dose of 50% Dextrose?

DIGOXIN   161–162

1. When is Digoxin indicated in the field?

2. How does Digoxin work to modify heart rate?

3. What is the usual dose and route of Digoxin?

4. When must caution be used for administering Digoxin?

5. What are the normal side effects of Digoxin?

6. What are the signs and symptoms of Digoxin toxicity?

7. What arrhythmias usually present with digitalis toxicity?

8. What is the pediatric dose of Digoxin?

DOPAMINE   162–163

1. What are the indications for Dopamine?

2. How does Dopamine work to increase blood pressure?

3. In addition to increasing blood pressure, what other actions does Dopamine have?

4. What is the dosage and route of Dopamine?

5. What major side effects can occur with Dopamine?

6. What clinical signs and symptoms are associated with infusing Dopamine too rapidly? Too slowly?

7. What complication can occur if the Dopamine drip infiltrates? What should be done then?

8. What is the pediatric dose of Dopamine?

EPINEPHRINE   163–164

1. Epinephrine 1:10,000 is used in the treatment of what conditions?

2. Epinephrine 1:1,000 is used in the treatment of what conditions?

3. What are the actions of Epinephrine on the heart? On the bronchial tree? On peripheral blood vessels?

4. How would you determine the effectiveness of Epinephrine?

5. What are the dosages, concentrations, and routes of administration of Epinephrine for treating cardiac arrhythmias? For asthma? For allergic reaction and anaphylaxis?

6. What are the possible side effects of Epinephrine?

7. Epinephrine should be used cautiously in treating patients with which conditions?

8. What is the drug of choice for treating asthmatics over 35 years of age?

9. What is the pediatric dose (including concentrations and routes) of Epinephrine for cardiac arrhythmias? For asthma? For allergic reactions and anaphylaxis?

GLUCAGON   164–165

1. When is Glucagon indicated?

2. What drug should be used if possible instead of Glucagon?

3. What are the actions of Glucagon?

4. What are the dosage and routes of Glucagon?

5. What procedure should be performed prior to administering Glucagon?

6. What are the side effects of Glucagon?

7. What are the effects of temperature on Glucagon, and what precautions should be taken in this regard?

8. What is the pediatric dose of Glucagon?

GLUCOLA   165

1. What is the field use of Glucola?

2. What is the action of Glucola?

3. What is the dosage range and route of administration of Glucola?

4. When is Glucola contraindicated?

5. How would you assess the patient's ability to swallow Glucola without aspirating?

6. What procedure should be performed prior to administering any glucose solution?

7. How is Glucola ordered in the pediatric patient?

INDERAL   166

1. When is Inderal indicated?

2. What are the actions of Inderal?

3. What is the dosage and route of Inderal?

4. When should Inderal be administered with caution?

5. What are the contraindications for use of Inderal?

6. What side effects can occur following administration of Inderal?

7. What is the pediatric dose of Inderal?

IPECAC   166–167

1. When is Ipecac indicated?

2. How does Ipecac work to induce vomiting?

3. What is the dosage and route of administration of Ipecac?

4. What clinical sign must be assessed prior to administering Ipecac?

5. Why is it important to dilute Ipecac with large amounts of clear fluids?

6. Ipecac is contraindicated in what types of ingested agents?

7. What is the pediatric dose of Ipecac?

ISUPREL   167–168

1. What are the primary indications for Isuprel?

2. How does Isuprel affect the heart? The respiratory system?

3. What is the dosage and route of administration of Isuprel for cardiac arrhythmias? For asthma?

4. What are the side effects of Isuprel?

5. What are the contraindications to the use of Isuprel?

6. With which drug does Isuprel have a cumulative effect?

7. In which patient group should Isuprel be used cautiously?

8. How is the effectiveness of Isuprel assessed in the cardiac patient? In the respiratory patient?

9. Patients who over-use an Isuprel inhaler might develop what condition?

LASIX   168–169

1. Lasix is used in the field treatment of what acute medical condition?

2. What are the actions of Lasix?

3. What is the dosage and route of administration of Lasix?

4. What is the major side effect of Lasix?

5. What is the contraindication for use of Lasix?

6. What physical parameters should be monitored to determine the effectiveness of Lasix?

7. Why is it important to report a patient's home use of diuretics?

8. What is the pediatric dose of Lasix?

LEVOPHED   169–170

1. What type of patient might require a Levophed drip?

2. How does Levophed work to increase blood pressure?

3. What are the dosage and route of administration of Levophed?

4. Which parameters must be monitored closely during Levophed administration?

5. What are the side effects of Levophed?

6. Why might you need to use atropine in conjunction with Levophed therapy?

7. What can happen if a Levophed drip infiltrates, and what should be done then?

8. What is the pediatric dose of Levophed?

LIDOCAINE   170–172

1. What are the indications for Lidocaine?

2. What is the action of Lidocaine?

3. What is the dosage and route of administration of Lidocaine for ventricular irritability? For prophylaxis against ventricular fibrillation?

4. What are the early and late signs of Lidocaine toxicity?

5. When is Lidocaine contraindicated?

6. Lidocaine should be used cautiously in patients with which disorder?

7. The dosage of Lidocaine should be reduced in the presence of which conditions?

8. What should be done at the first sign of Lidocaine toxicity?

9. What is the pediatric dose of Lidocaine?

MANNITOL   172

1. When is Mannitol indicated?

2. What are the actions of Mannitol?

3. What is the dosage and route of administration of Mannitol?

4. What is the major side effect of Mannitol?

5. Mannitol is contraindicated in which conditions?

6. What action must be taken if the Mannitol has crystalized in the bottle?

7. What is the pediatric dose of Mannitol?

METAPREL   172–173

1. What are the indications for Metaprel?

2. What is the action of Metaprel on the bronchial tree? On the heart?

3. What are the dosage and route of administration of Metaprel?

4. What are the side effects of Metaprel?

5. In which situation is Metaprel contraindicated?

6. How is the effectiveness of Metaprel determined?

7. What can happen from overuse of Metaprel?

8. In what situation should Metaprel be used cautiously?

9. What is the pediatric dose of Metaprel?

MORPHINE   173–174

1. What are the indications for Morphine?

2. What are the actions of Morphine?

3. What are the dosages and routes of administration of Morphine?

4. What are the side effects of Morphine?

5. What drug can be used to reverse the effects of Morphine?

6. What are the contraindications to use of Morphine?

7. What is the pediatric dose of Morphine?

NARCAN   174–175

1. What are the major uses of Narcan?

2. How does Narcan work?

3. What are the dosages and routes of administration of Narcan?

4. What are the side effects and contraindications of Narcan?

5. Against which drugs is Narcan effective?

6. Why is it important to monitor closely any patient to whom Narcan has been given?

7. What is the pediatric dose of Narcan?

NITROGLYCERINE   175–176

1. What are the indications for Nitroglycerine?

2. What are the actions of Nitroglycerine?

3. What is the dosage and route of administration of Nitroglycerine?

4. What are the side effects of Nitroglycerine?

5. What are the contraindications to use of Nitroglycerine?

6. What vital parameter must be assessed before and after administering Nitroglycerine?

7. What is the pediatric dose of Nitroglycerine?

NORMAL SALINE   176–177

1. What are the indications for using Normal Saline rather than another IV solution?

2. How does Normal Saline work?

3. How is Normal Saline administered?

4. When is Normal Saline contraindicated?

5. How is Normal Saline used in pediatric patients?

PITOCIN   177–178

1. When is Pitocin indicated?

2. How does Pitocin work?

3. What are the dosages and routes of administration of Pitocin?

4. What are the possible side effects of Pitocin?

5. When should Pitocin be used cautiously?

6. Why is Pitocin not administered prior to delivery of the infant and placenta?

7. What is the pediatric dose of Pitocin?

RINGER'S LACTATE   178–179

1. In which medical conditions is Ringer's indicated rather than another IV solution?

2. How does Ringer's work?

3. Why is a large bore cannula needle indicated when administering Ringer's?

4. When is Ringer's contraindicated?

5. In which patients should Ringer's be used with caution?

6. How is Ringer's administered to pediatric patients?

SODIUM BICARBONATE   179

1. What are the indications for use of Sodium Bicarbonate?

2. How does Sodium Bicarbonate work?

3. What are the dosages and route of administration of Sodium Bicarbonate?

4. What are the side effects and contraindications for Sodium Bicarbonate?

5. What condition results from over-administration of Sodium Bicarbonate?

6. What can occur with the administration of Sodium Bicarbonate to a well-ventilated patient?

7. What drug will precipitate when mixed with Sodium Bicarbonate?

8. What is the pediatric dose of Sodium Bicarbonate?

VALIUM   179–180

1. In which situations is Valium indicated?

2. How does Valium reduce seizure activity?

3. Why is Valium used before cardioverting?

4. What are the dosages and routes of administration of Valium?

5. What are the side effects of Valium?

6. When is Valium contraindicated?

7. In which conditions should Valium be used cautiously?

8. What can occur if IV Valium is administered too rapidly, and what action is then indicated?

9. When will IV Valium precipitate and how can this be prevented?

10. Valium has a cumulative effect with which agents?

11. What is the pediatric dose of Valium?

DRUG CALCULATIONS

CALCULATING DRUG DOSAGES

Once a drug order is received it is the paramedic's responsibility to administer that dosage as promptly and efficiently as possible. Unfortunately, drugs are rarely packaged in the exact dosage a patient needs. It is up to the paramedic to perform the necessary calculations to ensure that the patient receives the ordered dose. In the chaos of the emergency setting this task is a potential source of danger to the patient. To ensure patient safety, all paramedics must be as familiar with the arithmetic of drug calculations as they are with the pharmacology of the drugs themselves.

To become proficient in the area of drug calculations, paramedics must be able to perform safely in each of the following areas:

1. Equivalents of weights and measures.
2. Conversion from one unit of measure to others.
3. Calculating dosages for injection or oral administration.
4. Calculating drip rates for IV solutions.
5. Calculating dosages for IV drip medications.

The following pages contain the essential information required to make these necessary calculations, as well as examples of how the formulas are applied. Self-Assessment Questions are provided to test competency. The answers to the questions can be found at the end of the Drug Calculation section.

To avoid confusion in this section, the drops delivered by an IV set with a microdrop capacity (60 gtts/ml) will be referred to simply as drops, rather than microdrops. Since the capacity is always specified in the problem, the consistent use of gtts should clarify and simplify the required procedures.

1. EQUIVALENTS

WEIGHTS

1 kilogram (kg)	=	2.2 pounds (lb)
1 lb	=	16 ounces (oz)
30 grams (Gm)	=	1 oz
1 Gm	=	1000 mg
1 Gm	=	15 grains (gr)
60 mg	=	1 gr
1 mg	=	$\frac{1}{60}$ gr
1 mg	=	1000 micrograms (mcg)

MEASURES

1 liter (L)	=	1000 mililiters (ml)
1 quart (qt)	=	32 fluid ounces (fl oz)
1 L	=	1 qt
1 ml	=	1 cubic centimeter (cc)
500 ml	=	16 fl oz
250 ml	=	8 fl oz
30 ml	=	1 fl oz
15 ml	=	1 tablespoon (Tbsp)
1 teaspoon (tsp)	=	4–5 ml
1 ml	=	15 minims (m)

2. CONVERSIONS

Desired Conversion	Necessary Arithmetic	Example
mg to gr	divide mg by 60	300 mg ÷ 60 = 5 gr
gr to mg	muliply gr × 60	0.25 gr × 60 = 15 mg
lb to kg	divide lb by 2.2	77 lb ÷ 2.2 = 35 kg
kg to lb	multiply kg × 2.2	40 kg × 2.2 = 88 lb
mg to Gm	divide mg by 1000	6000 mg ÷ 1000 = 6 Gm
Gm to mg	multiply Gm × 1000	2 Gm × 1000 = 2000 mg
ml to Tbsp	divide ml by 15	45 ml ÷ 15 = 3 Tbsp
Tbsp to ml	multiply Tbsp × 15	6 Tbsp × 15 = 90 ml
ml to oz	divide ml by 30	30 ml ÷ 30 = 1 oz
oz to ml	multiply oz × 30	2 oz × 30 = 60 ml

3. CALCULATING DRUG DOSAGES FOR INJECTION OR ORAL ADMINISTRATION

Basic Formula

$$\frac{D \text{ (the amount DESIRED)}}{H \text{ (the amount you HAVE)}} = \text{The amount you should give}$$

SAMPLE PROBLEMS

1. You are to give 1 mg of atropine IV push. It comes in a concentration of 1 mg per 10 ml. How much do you give?
   SOLUTION:
   The amount desired is 1 mg. You have 1 mg in 10 ml.
   $$\frac{D}{H} = \frac{1 \text{ mg}}{1 \text{ mg/10 ml}} = 10 \text{ ml}$$
   You should give 10 ml.

2. You want to give 2.5 mg of Valium IV push. The syringe is marked 10 mg in 2 ml. How much do you give?
   SOLUTION: The amount desired is 2.5 mg. You have 10 mg. in 2 ml.
   $$\frac{D}{H} = \frac{2.5 \text{ mg}}{10 \text{ mg/2 ml}} = \frac{2.5 \text{ mg}}{5 \text{ mg/ml}} = \frac{2.5}{5 \text{ ml}} = 0.5 \text{ ml}$$
   You should give 0.5 ml

4. CALCULATING DRIP RATES FOR IV SOLUTIONS

Formula

$$\frac{\text{total volume ordered} \times \text{capacity of infusion set (gtts/ml)}^*}{\text{total time for infusion (in minutes)}} = \text{gtts/min}$$

*The capacity of IV infusion sets varies with manufacturer.
The gtts/ml for any specific tubing can be found on the package.

Example

You want to give 300 mg Aminophylline in 30 ml 5%DW via Volutrol over 30 minutes. The IV set you are using delivers 60 gtts/ml.
SOLUTION:

$$\frac{30 \text{ ml} \times 60 \text{ gtts/ml}}{30 \text{ min}} = \frac{1800 \text{ gtts}}{30 \text{ min}} = 60 \text{ gtts/min}$$

You should adjust the IV drip rate to 60 gtts/min.

5. CALCULATING DOSAGES FOR IV DRIP MEDICATIONS

Procedure

1. Convert to common units of measure
2. Determine number of mg in one ml of solution
3. Use D/H to determine ml/min
4. Multiply by the number of gtts/ml appropriate to the IV administration set

Example

You have 1 Gm Lidocaine in 500 ml 5%D/W. How many gtts/min do you need in order to deliver 1 mg/min of the Lidocaine?
SOLUTION:

1. Convert Gm to mg:
   1 Gm = 1000 mg
2. Find the number of mg in a single ml of solution:
   $$\frac{500 \text{ ml}}{1000 \text{ ml}} = 2 \text{ mg/ml}$$
3. Determine the number of ml/min required:
   $$\frac{D}{H} = \frac{1 \text{ mg/min}}{2 \text{ mg/ml}} = 0.5 \text{ ml/min}$$
4. Multiply the required ml/min by the number of gtts/ml delivered by the IV tubing being used:
   0.5 ml/min × 60 gtts/ml = 30 gtts/min
   You should infuse 30 gtts/min of solution to deliver 1 mg/min of Lidocaine.

SELF-ASSESSMENT QUESTIONS

1. You are ordered to add 1.5 mg Isuprel to 500 ml 5% D/W. You have Isuprel 5 mg in a 5 ml vial. How many mls do you add?

2. An MD ordered 30 ml Ipecac to be given to an overdose patient. How many tablespoons do you give?

3. You have 15 mg MS in a 1 ml vial. You are ordered to give ⅛ gr IM. How many mls do you administer?

4. Lasix comes in 2 ml amps containing 20 mg each. The order is for 100 mg IV. How many mls do you give?

5. You are ordered to give 250 mg Aminophylline IV Volutrol. You have 1 Gm in 10 ml. How many mls do you give?

6. You want to give 4 units Pitocin in an IV drip. You have a vial labeled 10 units per ml. How many mls do you add to the IV?

7. You are to give 500 mg calcium IV. You have 1 Gm in 10 ml. How many mls do you give?

8. You have 100 mg Lidocaine in a 10 ml preloaded syringe. Your order is for 75 mg. How many mls do you give?

9. You have a vial of atropine labeled 0.5 mg per ml. The patient needs a 1 mg bolus. How many mls do you give?

10. You are ordered to start an IV of Ringer's Lactate. Using IV tubing that delivers 10 gtts/cc, how fast would you set the rate to deliver each of the following volumes:
    a. 300 ml/hr
    b. 180 ml/hr
    c. 500 ml/hr
    d. 250 ml/hr

11. You are ordered to give 250 mg Aminophylline in 20 ml 5% D/W over 30 minutes via Volutrol drip. You have 250 mg Aminophylline in 10 ml. Your IV set delivers 60 gtts/ml. How fast should you set the drip rate to infuse the 30 ml contained in the Volutrol?

12. You are ordered to start an IV of RL as a precautionary measure in an asymptomatic trauma patient. Your administration set delivers 10 gtts/ml. How fast should you set the drip rate to deliver 30 ml/hr?

13. You are ordered to prepare a Lidocaine drip to control PVCs. Using an IV set that delivers 60 gtts/ml, calculate the number of gtts/min that you would use to infuse each of the following:
    a. 1 Gm in 250 ml at 4 mg/min
    b. 2 Gm in 500 ml at 2 mg/min
    c. 2 Gm in 250 ml at 4 mg/min

14. The maximum amount of Lidocaine that can safely be infused over one hour is 4 mg/kg. Your patient weighs 176 lbs. You have prepared

an IV drip of 2 Gm Lidocaine in 500 ml 5% D/W.

   a. What is the maximum amount of Lidocaine this patient can receive in one hour?

   b. How many mg/ml are there in the mixture you have prepared?

   c. Assume you have already given a 100 mg bolus of Lidocaine. Subtracting that, how much more Lidocaine can safely be administered over one hour?

   d. You are ordered to run your drip at 3 mg/min. Does this exceed the safe rate of 4 mg/kg/hr?

ANSWERS TO SELF-ASSESSMENT QUESTIONS

  1. 1.5 ml
  2. 2 Tbsp
  3. 0.5 ml
  4. 10 ml
  5. 2.5 ml
  6. 0.4 ml
  7. 5 ml
  8. 7.5 ml
  9. 2 ml
10a. 50 gtts/min
  b. 30 gtts/min
  c. 83 gtts/min
  d. 42 gtts/min
11. 60 gtts/min
12. 5 gtts/min
13a. 60 gtts/min
  b. 30 gtts/min
  c. 30 gtts/min
14a. 320 mg
  b. 4 mg/ml
  c. 220 mg
  d. no, it is a safe rate

COMMON HOME MEDICATIONS

INTRODUCTION

Many times, the only clue you will have to the possible cause of the patient's problem will be a handful of prescription drugs found in the home. Sometimes the kinds of medications a person is taking will help to suggest a possible diagnosis. The following are categories of drugs commonly found in the home. Each summary gives a brief description of the uses and actions of these agents, as well as a sampling of some of the more common medications included in that category.

Analgesics

Analgesics are drugs that reduce pain. They can accomplish this in one or more of the following ways:

- raising the threshold of pain
- diminishing local response to pain
- altering the psychologic response to pain
- alleviating anxiety and apprehension

The amount of pain a person experiences will vary from time to time depending upon the patient's physical and emotional status, and will differ between individuals. Analgesics are not normally prescribed unless an attempt has been made to treat the cause of the pain, but often a patient is sent home on some type of analgesic to control pain during the treatment process. The type of analgesic ordered will depend largely on the cause of the pain as well as on its location and severity.

Aspirin (ASA)
Aspirin, Phenacetin, and
    Caffeine (APC's)
Bufferin
Cocaine
Darvocet-N
Darvon
Darvon compound
Demerol
Dilaudid

Empirin with Codeine #3 (30 mg)
Fiorinal
Heroin
Methadone
Percodan
Percogesic
Phenaphen
Talwin
Tylenol with Codeine #3, #4

Home Medications

Anorexiants

Commonly called "diet pills," anorexiants are drugs that are given to control the appetite, usually to help the patient lose weight. The most common of these are the amphetamine or amphetamine-like drugs that have a tendency to produce psychic, and occasionally physical, dependency on the drug. Because of this side effect, most physicians now prefer to give nutritional guidance and psychologic counseling rather than prescribing these agents. The original explanation of the action of anorexiants suggested that they stimulate the central nervous system (CNS); this theory was discarded after recent studies showed that they actually affect the control center in the hypothalamus. These drugs will cause anorexia, but they also produce an increase in awareness, initiative, and motor activity, which contributes to a decreased sensation of fatigue.

Amphetamine (Benzedrine)	**Preludin**
Dexadrine	**Pre-Sate**
Didrex	**Ritalin**
Ionamin	**Tenuate (Tepanil)**
Opatrol	**Wilpo**
Plegine	

Antacids

Antacids are agents used to reduce the acidity of the stomach and duodenum. They are particularly useful in controlling the symptoms of peptic ulcers, gastritis, indigestion, and other disorders of the upper gastrointestinal tract. By raising the pH of the stomach to 5.0, many of the adverse effects of hyperacidity can be greatly reduced.

Alka Seltzer	**PeptoBismol**
Amphojel	**Riopan**
DiGel	**Rolaids**
Gaviscon	**Sodium bicarbonate**
Gelusil	**Tums**
Maalox	
Mylanta	

Antianginal Agents

Antianginal agents were originally labeled coronary vasodilators because they were thought to relieve angina by dilating coronary blood vessels. We now know that they also dilate the periphery to a small degree, thereby easing the workload of the heart and reducing the myocardial oxygen requirements.

Amyl nitrate	Nitranitol
Cardilate	Nitrobid Paste
Inderal	Nitroglycerine
Isordil (sorbitrate)	Peritrate

Antiarrhythmics

As their name suggests, these agents are used to control the rhythm of the heart and prevent arrhythmias that could endanger the patient. These drugs are commonly prescribed following any kind of cardiac insult that would potentially produce rhythm disturbances. Such conditions include myocardial infarction, open heart surgery, pericarditis, congestive heart failure, and valvular disease.

Dilantin (ventricular arrhythmias)	Pronestyl (ventricular arrhythmias)
Inderal (supraventricular & ventricular arrhythmias)	Quinaglute (supraventricular & ventricular arrhythmias)
Lanoxin (supraventricular)	Quinidine (supraventricular & ventricular arrhythmias)
Norpase (supraventricular and ventricular)	

Antibiotics

Antibiotics are in widespread use to combat specific bacteria and other microorganisms once a culture is read to identify the cause. Certain strains of organisms become immune to the agents and require different drugs or dosing. Underdosing can result in recurrence of certain infections, while overdosing can result in severe diarrhea and nausea. These drugs frequently produce allergic reactions, particularly Penicillin and the sulfonamides.

Ampicillin	Kantrex (kanamycin)
Ancef	Keflex
Azogantrisin	Macrodantin
Azogantonol	Mandelamine
Azulfadine	Nafcillin
Bactrim	NegGram
Chloramphenicol	Oxacillin
Cleocin	Penicillin
Dicloxacillin	Septra
Duracef	Streptomycin
Erythromycin	Sulfamylon acetate (mafenide acetate)
Furadantin	

| Gantanol | Tetracycline |
| Gantrisin | Vibramycin |

Anticoagulants

Anticoagulants act by prolonging the prothrombin time which produces a delay in blood clotting. These agents are essential in preventing thrombosis formation associated with various cardiovascular diseases and following various cardiac and orthopedic operations. Patients sent home on oral anticoagulants are cautioned regarding the use of aspirin which can affect clotting. They are also instructed to watch for excessive bleeding and to have periodic laboratory studies to ensure they are on the right maintenance dose.

| Coumadin (warfarin) | Heparin for injection |
| Dicumarol | Sintrom |

Anticonvulsants

Anticonvulsant agents act by raising the threshold for cerebral irritation without greatly incapacitating the patient. The agents and the dosages are varied according to the type of seizures present and the patient status. They may be prescribed acutely or on a maintenance dose for life. Side effects and/or overdosing can inhibit fine motor coordination and therefore can limit the activities of those patients who require high doses for seizure control.

Dilantin (Phenytoin)	Mysoline
Phenobarbital	Tegretol
Mebaral	Tridione
Mephenytoin (mesantoin)	Zarontin

Antidepressants

A common psychiatric problem requiring drug therapy is depression. The two most common classifications of antidepressants currently in use have different pharmacologic action. *Tricyclic compounds* potentiate the adrenergic effects by preventing the uptake of norepinephrine within the central nervous system. Severe tachyarrhythmias may occur from an overdose of these agents and may require Physostigmine or even defibrillation. *Monoamine oxidase (MAO) inhibitors* prevent impulse transmissions at the synapse between neurons and also may interrupt catecholamine breakdown. If the patient accidentally combines narcotics with MAO inhibitors or overdoses on MAO inhibitors, cardiac irritability may occur.

Tricyclic Compounds
    Adapin (Sinequan)
    Aventyl
    Elavil
    Norpramin (Pertofrane)
    Tofranil
    Triavil
    Vivactil

MAO Inhibitors
    Marplan
    Nardil
    Parnate

Antidiarrheal Agents

Diarrhea may occur either chronically or acutely as a result of various drugs, infections, allergies or ischemic conditions. Specific agents which are used to restore the bowel's normal motility and absorption are listed below. Overdose of these drugs can result in paralytic ileus, with the patient complaining of severe abdominal pain.

Bacid (Lactinex)	Kaolin with pectin
Bismuth Salts	Kaopectate
Cantil	Lomotil
Donnagel PG	Paregoric
Flagyl	Parepectolin
Furoxone	Sorboquel

Antiemetic Agents

Antiemetic agents are used to prevent or relieve nausea and vomiting. These agents are very useful in patients with motion sickness or middle ear infections. Antiemetics are also used to counteract the nausea and vomiting which are caused by chemotherapy used to treat cancer patients. Oral preparations and rectal suppositories are often the prescribed routes of administration for home use. Drowsiness is a very common side effect of antiemetic agents because of their associated sedative action.

Atarax	Tigan
Compazine	Thorazine
Dramamine	Torecan
Emetecon	Vistaril
Phenergan	

Antihistamines

Antihistamine agents help prevent further release of histamine in an allergic reaction, thus helping to suppress associated signs and symptoms.

They are used for hay fever and urticaria but are of little value in preventing an acute asthma or allergic attack. Antihistamines have an associated sedative effect, so use in conjunction with alcohol or CNS depressants can cause a decreased level of consciousness or respiratory depression.

Benadryl	**Phenergan**
Chlor-Trimeton (Histaspan,	**Pribenzamine HCL**
Teldrin)	**Pyribenzamine citrate**
Clistin	**Pyrilamine maleate**
Decapryn	**Temaril**
Dimetane	**Triten**
Disomer	**Vistaril (Atarax)**
Histadyl	
Periactin	

Antihypertensive Agents

Antihypertensive agents are usually used in combination with other drugs such as diuretics and sedatives to lower and maintain the patient's blood pressure to a diastolic of 100 or below. Most antihypertensive drugs work by causing vasodilatation in the periphery. A common side effect of antihypertensive therapy is hypotension.

Aldomet (Methyldopa)	**Ismelin**
Apresoline	**Lopressor**
Corgard	**Minipres**
Catapres	**Minizide**
Diamox	**Serapes**
Inderal	**Serpasil (Reserpine)**
Inversine	

Antipsychotic Agents

Antipsychotic agents are major tranquilizers that are prescribed to alter the symptoms of acute and chronic behavioral disorders resulting from mental illness. In therapeutic doses, these medications enable the individual to cope with his/her illness and function in the activities of daily living, without producing the stuporous side effects of most sedatives. Since mental illness is a widespread affliction in today's society, you may encounter many patients on these medications.

Phenothiazine Agents:	**Thioxanthine Agents:**
Mellaril	**Haldol**
Prolixin (Permitil)	**Lithane (Eskalith, Lithonate)**

Serentil	Navane
Sparine	Taractan
Stelazine	
Thorazine	
Trilafon	
Vesprin	

Antispasmodics

Antispasmodics are used to relieve the pain associated with excessive gastrointestinal smooth muscle contractions. These agents are used in GI disorders such as colitis. They work by blocking acetylcholine in the parasympathetic nervous system. Antispasmodics very often produce associated central nervous system depression.

Banthine	Librax
Belladonna extracts	Pro-Banthine
Bentyl	Robinul
Donnatal	

Antituberculosis Agents

During the last 25 years there has been a sharp decline in the incidence of tuberculosis due to the use of chemotherapeutic agents. Antituberculosis drugs work against this inflammatory, communicable disease by deactivating the tubercle bacillus. Tuberculosis commonly attacks the lungs but may be found in any part of the body.

The drugs listed are frequently used concurrently for a more therapeutic effect.

Ethambutol	Rifampin
Isoniazid (INH)	Streptomycin (SM)
Paraminosalicylic acid (PAS)	

Bronchodilators

Bronchodilators act by relaxing the smooth muscles of the bronchioles and are beneficial in controlling bronchospasm associated with chronic pulmonary diseases such as asthma, bronchitis and emphysema. Most COPD patients are on some form of bronchodilator medications at home. Bronchodilators may be taken orally, by aerosol inhalers, and occasionally by suppository.

Aminophylline	Metraprel (alupent)
Bronkosol	Quibron
Bronkotabs	Slophyllin

Isuprel Mistometer   Tedral
LãBid   Terbutaline
Marax

Cardiac Glycosides

Cardiac glycosides are digitalis preparations that are frequently prescribed for the management of chronic congestive heart failure and for the control of certain rhythm disturbances, specifically atrial fibrillation and atrial flutter. They act to improve myocardial contractility by increasing stroke volume and slowing the conduction through the SA and AV nodes. This improves cardiac output by allowing the ventricles to rest and fill more completely between contractions. Digitalis preparations also cause the heart to pump more efficiently and reduce myocardial oxygen consumption. Patients are commonly placed on digitalis preparations following myocardial infarction or acute episodes of congestive heart failure. When antiarrhythmic agents such as quinidine, Pronestyl, or Inderal are simultaneously prescribed, you should suspect that the patient had a previous myocardial infarction and anticipate arrhythmias.

Digitalis toxicity occurs occasionally in patients taking digitalis preparations and may be the reason you are called to the scene. Despite the frequent and early occurrences of gastrointestinal symptoms indicating digitalis toxicity, a disturbance of cardiac rhythm is usually the first evidence of toxicity. Frequently occurring arrhythmias include PVCs, first degree AV block, sinus arrest, SA block, atrial tachycardia with block, ventricular bigeminy, and even ventricular tachycardia. Other signs of toxicity include anorexia and visual disturbances such as diplopia, halo effect around dark objects, or a yellow or green tinge to objects.

Gitaligin   Digoxin (Lanoxin)
Digitoxin   Digitalis leaf

Diuretics

Patients are placed on oral diuretic agents at home to control the edema that frequently accompanies chronic congestive heart failure or renal insufficiency. Diuretics act by stimulating the kidneys to excrete excess water and sodium, usually by inhibiting the reabsorption of sodium at the renal tubules. Since potassium is excreted along with sodium and water, these patients are usually on concurrent potassium supplements. Excessive serum potassium depletion or elevation can induce ventricular arrhythmias.

Aquatag (Edemex)   Hydrodiuril (hydrochlorathiazide,
Aquatensen   HCTZ, Esidrex, Oretic)

Aldactazide
Aldactone
Anhydron
Dyazide
Diuril
Edecrin (ethacrinic acid)

Hydromox
Hygroton
Lasix
Naqua (Metahydrin)
Naturetin
Saluron
Triamterene

Hormones

Hormones are complex chemical agents manufactured by the body's endocrine glands to control growth, sexual development, metabolism, and electrolyte balance. Occasionally a deficiency can occur which may require treatment by the administration of natural or synthetic hormones. Most oral contraceptives contain hormones. Hormone therapy has also been used to combat certain carcinomas.

Amnestrogen (Evex, Menest)
Diethylstilbestrol
Estradiol (Aquadiol, Delestrogen)
Estrone (Ogen, Femspan)
Gesterol
Hexadrol
Meprane

Nelalutin
Premarin
Provera, Depo-Provera
Synestrol
Tace
Vallestril

Common Oral Contraceptives:

Demulen
Enovid
Norinyl
Norlestrin
Norquen

Oracon
Ortho-Novum
Ovral
Ovulen

Hypoglycemic Agents

Hypoglycemic agents are used to control diabetes mellitus. This is a hereditary disease which results when the body is unable to metabolize glucose properly. These agents may be injected or taken orally, and the dosage varies according to the patient's health, diet, and exercise routine. Diabetics usually adjust their own medications, and occasionally they miscalculate, leading to hyper- or hypoglycemic states.

Insulins for injection:
Crystalline zinc
Lente
NPH

Oral hypoglycemics:
Diabinese
Dymelor
Orinase

Regular (short-acting)   Tolbutamide
                                          Tolinase

Laxatives and Stool Softeners

Laxatives and stool softeners are drugs that prevent constipation by
generally altering fecal consistency and by stimulating peristalsis. They
are dispensed in oral, liquid or suppository form and can be either prescribed or purchased "over the counter."

Most elderly or confined individuals are on some form of daily laxative,
as inactivity contributes to constipation. Patients with gastrointestinal
disorders may take these medications to control their condition.

Cascara	Metamucil
Castor oil	Milk of Magnesia (MOM)
Colace	Mineral oil
Dulcolax	Pericolace
Glycerin suppositories	Senakot

Sedatives and Hypnotics

Sedatives are central nervous system depressants used to calm nervousness, irritability, and excitement. Hypnotics are agents which are used to
induce sleep. Both groups of these drugs may be abused and can lead to
respiratory depression, coma, and death.

Sedatives:

Librium	Valium
Phenobarbital	Thorazine

Hypnotics:

Chloral hydrate	Placidyl
Dalmane	Phenobarbital
Equanil (Miltown)	Quaalude (methaqualone)
Nembutal (pentobarbital)	Tuinal
Noludar	Seconal (secobarbital)

Steroids

Steroids are effective in treating chronic adrenocortical insufficiency,
allergic reactions, collagen disorders, and other inflammatory processes.
Although the method by which steroids control inflammatory processes is
not fully understood, they have a wide spectrum of application. Patients on
steroid therapy may experience mild GI bleeding and a diminished resistance to infection. If patients are not being closely managed, they may

suffer an adrenocortical crisis, especially when being weaned off steroids. A controlled, gradual weaning will allow the body to adjust to the decreased level of circulating steroids.

Celestone

Cortisone acetate

Dexamethasone (Decadron, Hexadrol)

Florinef acetate

Hydrocortisone

Prednisolone

Prednisone

Solu-Cortef

Solu-Medrol

SECTION III:
ARRHYTHMIA
INTERPRETATION

CONTENTS

INTRODUCTION

This section is designed to review the basic principles of electrocardiography and arrhythmia interpretation. It is not a substitute for a course in electrocardiography. Arrhythmia interpretation is often difficult and should only be approached if you have had actual training in interpreting EKGs, since inexperienced persons can easily become confused and develop misconceptions that are difficult to correct.

The EKG section has been organized to review arrhythmias in a systematic manner. First, there is a general review of electrophysiology and the principles of electrocardiography. Following this, each of the most common arrhythmias is discussed in order of its occurrence within the conduction system. Each profile contains a summary of etiology, identifying EKG features, clinical picture, and treatment of these types of cardiac problems.

The discussion of common arrhythmias is followed by a brief description of several electrocardiographic phenomenon which may confuse or modify your interpretation of arrhythmias. These include such topics as bundle branch block and ST changes.

Finally, there is a self-assessment section which includes questions on basic principles as well as a variety of patient situations which require arrhythmia interpretation and management. All of the EKG strips in this section should be interpreted as being Lead II.

In utilizing this section for review, avoid the temptation to use pattern recognition of EKG strips. Instead, visualize and understand the physiologic activity within the heart that produced the arrhythmia and the expected clinical manifestations. Use a consistent organized approach to gather all the information available from the EKG and compare it to the identifying features listed for each arrhythmia prior to your interpretation. The rates quoted for the various arrhythmias are to be used solely as guidelines for clinical interpretation of the EKG strip, and should not be considered inflexible standards.

All cardiac arrhythmias should be evaluated for their effect on cardiac output or their potential for progression to a lethal arrhythmia. Determine the required treatment by assessing the patient thoroughly, as well as identifying the arrhythmia.

Begin this section by reviewing all of the basic EKG principles, then answer the questions and approach the clinical situations. After you have completed the Self-Assessment section, turn to the answer key and compare it to your own interpretations and treatments. Concentrate on weak areas and seek additional help from your instructor or medical personnel in your paramedic program until you are comfortable with your knowledge of arrhythmias.

ELECTROPHYSIOLOGY

Electrophysiology

The heart is composed of two types of cells which enable it to perform two distinct functions:

Electrical: Specialized cells which make up the conduction system and have the specific ability to initiate and transmit electrical activity in the heart.

Mechanical: Myocardial cells which make up the bulk musculature of the heart and contract in response to electrical stimuli.

The electrical impulse is responsible for stimulating the heart's mechanical contraction and is necessary for the heart to pump effectively. Although arrhythmias affect mechanical activity, they are caused by malfunctions in the electrical system. Therefore, in order to understand arrhythmias it is vital to understand the normal conduction system and how it works. The physical layout of the heart's electrical conduction system is diagrammed in Figure 3.1.

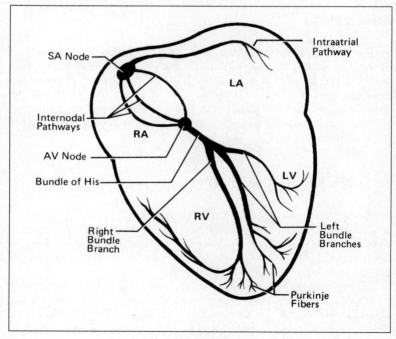

Figure 3.1

215

Electrical activity begins in the sinoatrial (SA) node and flows toward the ventricles. All areas of the conduction system have the ability to 1) initiate impulses, 2) respond to impulses, and 3) become irritable.

Each area of the conduction system initiates impulses at its own inherent rate as shown here:

SA Node   60–100 times per minute
AV Junction   40–60 times per minute
Ventricle   20–40 times per minute

In general, the fastest pacemaker site will predominate and determine the heart rate. The SA node is the usual pacemaker site since it initiates impulses at a faster rate than the junction or ventricle. However, if for some reason the SA node should fail, an impulse from the AV junction can *"escape"* and take over to pace the heart. Likewise, if the junction also fails, the ventricles can then take over. This protective backup system helps maintain the heart's electrical efficiency. There are times, however, when the junction or the ventricle becomes *irritable* and initiates impulses at a faster than normal rate, thus overriding the SA node and taking over control of the heart.

Innervation

Heart rate and myocardial contractility are influenced by the autonomic nervous system (ANS) via *sympathetic* and/or *parasympathetic* stimulation. Normal function is dependent on the proper balance of these two systems. However, if one or the other is either stimulated or blocked, the balance will be disrupted, resulting in abnormal function of the conduction system and subsequent arrhythmias. The ANS control of the heart is outlined in Figure 3.2.

Graphic Display of EKG

The electrical forces within the heart can be detected by electrodes attached to the patient's skin. If the flow of current is *toward* the positive electrode, the graphic display will depict a positive or upright mark on the EKG paper. If the flow is *away from* the positive electrode, the EKG deflection will be negative, or downward.

Since the main flow of electrical activity in the heart travels from the SA node to the ventricles, the current is normally moving toward the positive electrode in Lead II. This produces a primarily upright complex with clearly visible P waves, which makes Lead II a valuable monitoring lead.

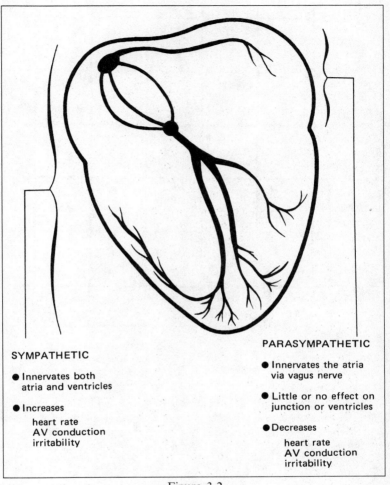

SYMPATHETIC

● Innervates both
   atria and ventricles

● Increases

   heart rate
   AV conduction
   irritability

PARASYMPATHETIC

● Innervates the atria
   via vagus nerve

● Little or no effect on
   junction or ventricles

● Decreases

   heart rate
   AV conduction
   irritability

Figure 3.2

The basis for EKG interpretation is the use of a consistent medium for producing the written display of electrical activity. To serve this purpose, all EKG graph paper is uniform in its markings and the speed of the EKG machine or oscilloscope is standardized. By matching the markings made by the patient's electrical activity to the time and voltage measures on the graph paper, you can calculate the measurements of the patient's complex and compare them to "normal" or to the patient's preillness state. Standard graph paper measurements are shown in Figure 3.3 (p. 218).

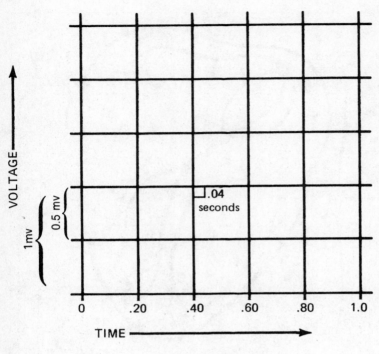

Figure 3.3

As the heart generates electrical impulses, each will create a distinct pattern on the graph paper. Each deflection has normal boundaries and an identifying definition to help isolate it, and subsequently to identify the causative electrical activity. These definitions are outlined in Figure 3.4.

Electrical Activity	Associated Pattern	Graphic Depiction
Atrial Depolarization	P Wave	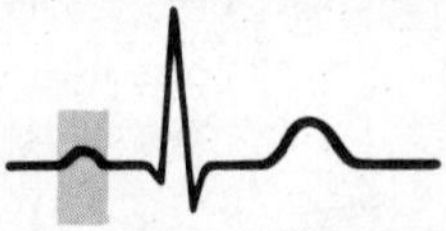
Delay at AV Node	PR Segment	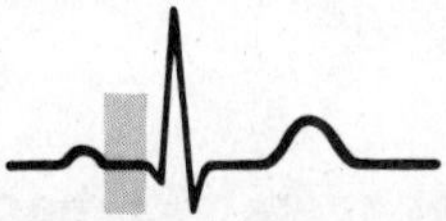
Ventricular Depolarization	QRS Complex	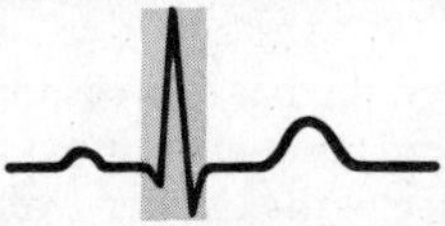
Ventricular Repolarization	T Wave	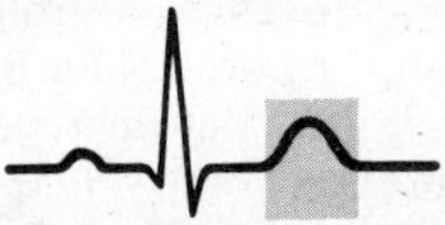
No electrical activity	Isoelectric Line	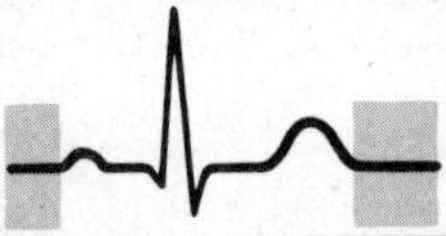

Figure 3.4

Each electrical pacemaker impulse produces a cardiac cycle on the EKG, and in a healthy heart the mechanical cells will respond by producing a cardiac contraction. If the mechanical system is functioning effectively, you should be able to feel a pulse beat with each cardiac cycle. However, if the EKG shows a normal cardiac cycle which you'd expect to produce a pulse, but no pulse is present, suspect a malfunction of the heart's mechanical system. The correlation between cardiac cycles on the EKG and the patient's pulse beats is shown in Figure 3.5 (p. 220).

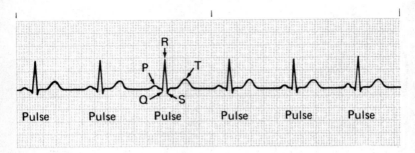

Figure 3.5

Electrical Refractoriness

When the heart is responding actively to an electrical stimulus, it cannot accept another stimulus and is totally unresponsive, or "refractory." This phase of the cardiac cycle is called the *absolute* refractory period (ARP). Refractoriness is a protective mechanism that prevents the heart from responding to all of the impulses fired by an excessively rapid pacemaker.

At the end of the repolarization phase, some of the cells will recover before others and will be able to accept a new impulse if it is strong enough. This phase is called the *relative* refractory period (RRP). Both refractory periods are illustrated in Figure 3.6.

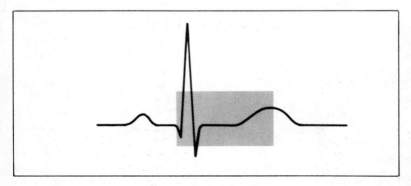

Figure 3.6

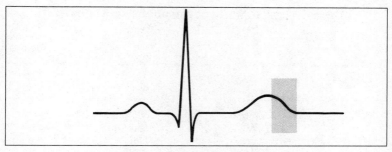

Relative Refractory Period

If a strong stimulus falls during the relative refractory period, it may depolarize some of the cells while others remain refractory. This "sloppy" discharge can cause sudden ventricular irritability, including arrhythmias such as ventricular tachycardia or ventricular fibrillation. Therefore, the relative refractory period is called the vulnerable phase of the cardiac cycle and becomes important if ventricular ectopics begin to occur on or near the T wave.

Approach to Arrhythmia Interpretation

When analyzing an arrhythmia, you must be able to identify the electrical activity within the heart that produced the pattern. It isn't as important to be able to name the arrhythmia as it is to understand its mechanism and its effect on the patient. For this reason, it is vitally important that you avoid the temptation to use pattern recognition of arrythmias. Instead, develop a consistent method for approaching rhythm strips and employ it with every arrhythmia you interpret. You will soon find yourself using it automatically, and only thinking of it consciously when you come to a difficult arrhythmia.

When analyzing an arrhythmia, ask yourself what's happening within that heart. The rate and rhythm will give you some idea of the effectiveness of the pattern and the impact it will have on the patient's cardiac output. Next, locate each of the P waves, then the QRS complexes. Evaluate the relationship between them as shown by the PR intervals (PRIs). This should explain the interrelation of atrial activity to ventricular activity. Don't forget to look at your patient and assess perfusion; remember, when it comes time to treat, it is the patient who receives the drug, not the EKG strip. An example of an organized approach to arrhythmia interpretation is shown in Table 3.1

Table 3.1 Systematic Approach to Arrhythmia Interpretation

	Questions to ask	Things to consider
Rhythm:	Is it regular? Is it irregular? Are there any early beats? Are there any late beats?	If the R-R interval varies less than .04–.08 sec, it can be considered regular.
Rate:	What is the exact rate? Is it normal? Is it rapid? Is it slow? Is the atrial rate the same as the ventricular rate?	Rates are merely guidelines. Rates will frequently affect cardiac output and cause symptoms
P wave:	Is it present or not? Is the shape normal? Is it upright in Lead II? Is there one P for every QRS? Is the P in front of the QRS or behind it? Are there more Ps than QRSs? Do all the Ps look alike? Where are the dissimilar P waves?	The P wave is often the key to diagnosing the arrhythmia. If it's normal, the arrhythmia is of sinus origin. If it's flattened or otherwise unusual, it's atrial. If it's inverted, it's junctional. If it's absent, it could be atrial, junctional, or ventricular.
PR interval:	What is the PRI? Is it normal? Is it prolonged? Are all the PRIs constant? If the PRI is not constant is it getting longer?	If it's constant, there is conduction through the AV node If it varies, there is an AV disturbance. If it's longer than normal, there is delay in the AV node If there is no relation, they are dissociated

| *QRS complex:* | What is the QRS?
Is it of normal duration?
Is it wider than normal?
Do they all look alike?
Does it have a normal
relationship to the P? | If it's narrow, the ar-
rhythmia is supraventricu-
lar.
If it's wider than .12 it's
probably ventricular;
sometimes supraventricu-
lar arrhythmias have a
wide QRS. |

Calculating Heart Rate

There are several methods by which you can calculate the heart rate from an EKG tracing. All are based on the fact that the vertical lines on the EKG graph paper are spaced .04 seconds apart. By measuring the R-R interval you can calculate the ventricular rate, while the P-P interval will measure the atrial rate. Both rates should be calculated on each rhythm strip to identify any differences in atrial and ventricular activity. Three methods of calculating heart rate are shown in Table 3.2.

Table 3.2   Calculating Heart Rates

Method	Features
1500 divided by the number of small squares between 2 R waves	• most accurate • only used with regular rhythms • Takes time to figure
No. of R waves in 6 sec. x 10	• very inaccurate • only good for irregular rhythms • very quick estimate
300 divided by the number of large squares between 2 R waves or	• very quick • not very accurate with fast rates • only used with regular rhythms

Memorize This Scale

1 large square	=	300 beats/min
2 " "	=	150 beats/min
3 " "	=	100 beats/min
4 " "	=	75 beats/min
5 " "	=	60 beats/min
6 " "	=	50 beats/min

COMMON ARRHYTHMIAS

NORMAL SINUS RHYTHM

Etiology

Normal sinus rhythm (NSR) refers to the normal electrical pattern of the heart. In this rhythm, the SA node is the pacemaker and initiates electrical impulses which follow normal pathways and travel within normal time frames.

Identifying Features

Rhythm: regular
Rate: 60–100 beats/min
P wave: normal and upright in Lead II
PRI: .12–.20 seconds and constant
QRS: less than .12 seconds

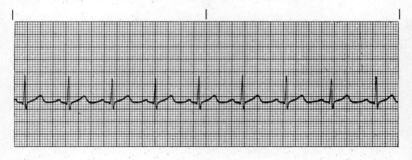

Clinical Picture

Does not produce symptoms.

Treatment

Does not require treatment.

SINUS TACHYCARDIA

Etiology

In sinus tachycardia (ST), the SA node is the pacemaker and discharges impulses at a rate greater than 100 beats/minute. Conduction through the atria and ventricles is normal. The increased rate can be attributed to overactivity of the sympathetic nervous system or blocking of the parasympathetic nervous system. This may be caused by fever, anxiety, pain, or physical activity. Sinus tachycardia may also be an attempt to compensate for a drop in cardiac output.

Identifying Features

Rhythm: regular
Rate: greater than 100, usually 100–160 beats/min
P wave: normal and upright in Lead II
PRI: .12–.20 seconds and constant
QRS: less than .12 seconds

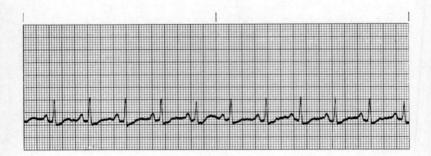

Clinical Picture

- rapid regular pulse
- patient may complain of palpitations or dyspnea, or may be asymptomatic
- in the presence of an MI, may extend the infarction or induce CHF due to increased myocardial workload and oxygen consumption

Treatment

To treat this arrhythmia correctly you must identify the underlying cause by thorough history and physical exam and treat accordingly. It is not sufficient merely to slow the heart rate by vagotonic maneuvers and medications.

SINUS BRADYCARDIA

Etiology

In sinus bradycardia (SB), the SA node is the pacemaker and discharges impulses at a rate of less than 60 beats per minute. Conduction follows the normal pathways. This slow rate is usually caused by increased parasympathetic (vagal) influence on the SA node. Other possible causes for a bradycardia include SA node damage, hypoxia, and drug overdose. Athletes frequently develop this arrhythmia as a result of prolonged physical conditioning.

Identifying Features

Rhythm: regular
Rate: less than 60 beats/min
P wave: normal and upright in Lead II
PRI: .12–.20 seconds and constant
QRS: less than .12 seconds

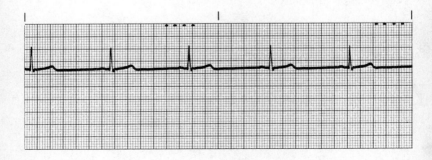

Clinical Picture

- slow, regular pulse
- does not usually produce signs or symptoms of decreased cardiac output
- if rate is markedly slow, the decreased blood flow can lead to syncope or angina
- can be a warning of potential dangers such as blocks or asystole
- the slow rate can precipitate escape rhythms or ventricular irritability

Treatment

If the patient develops signs or symptoms of decreased cardiac output or ventricular irritability, treat the arrhythmia by increasing the heart rate. This is usually accomplished with atropine. Remember, PVCs associated with a bradycardia are *not* treated with Lidocaine.

SINUS ARRHYTHMIA

Etiology

In sinus arrhythmia, the SA node continues to be the pacemaker but discharges impulses at irregular intervals. This irregularity is caused by fluctuations in vagal activity during respiration. Heart rate increases with each inspiration and decreases with each expiration. This arrhythmia is very common in children.

Identifying Features

Rhythm: irregular
Rate: usually 60–100 beats/min
P wave: normal and upright in Lead II
PRI: .12–.20 seconds and constant
QRS: less than .12 seconds

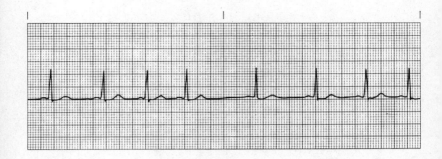

Clinical Picture

- irregular pulse

Treatment

Does not require treatment.

PREMATURE ATRIAL CONTRACTIONS

Etiology

A premature atrial contraction (PAC) occurs when an irritable focus in the atrium initiates an impulse which temporarily overrides the SA node. These premature beats can be distinguished from normal sinus beats because they occur early in the cardiac cycle and have a P wave of different morphology than the sinus beats, i.e., peaked, flattened, notched, diphasic, or hidden in the T wave. PACs usually have normal conduction through the AV node and the ventricles. Atrial irritability is often indicative of myocardial damage, hypoxia, or drug overdose.

Identifying Features

Rhythm: underlying rhythm will be interrupted by early beat

Rate: depends on underlying arrhythmia

P wave: P wave of early beat differs from sinus beat, or may be lost in T wave

PRI: .12–.20 seconds (may be prolonged due to AV node refractoriness)

QRS: less than .12 seconds

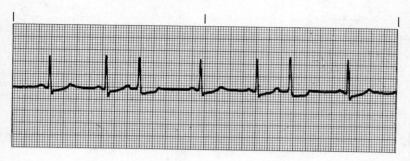

Clinical Picture

- irregular pulse
- patient is unaware of premature beats but they may be detected by palpating a pulse or auscultating the heart
- positive identification can only be made by EKG

Treatment

Isolated PACs are of minimal significance and very often are corrected by oxygen alone. However, frequent PACs may be an early indication of CHF and may lead to atrial tachyarrhythmias. Therefore, watch patient closely and treat the underlying cause of the PACs if indicated.

ATRIAL TACHYCARDIA

Etiology

In atrial tachycardia, an irritable focus within the atrium supresses activity of the SA node by initiating impulses at a rate of 150–250 beats/minute. Each impulse is conducted to the ventricles. The atrial P waves appear to be identical, but they do vary in morphology from the sinus P wave because they arise from a different focus. They may be peaked, flattened, notched, diphasic, or hidden in the T wave. If the P waves cannot be identified and ventricular conduction is normal, the arrhythmia is then loosely described as a supraventricular tachycardia because it cannot be distinguished from other supraventricular arrhythmias in the same rate range. Atrial tachycardia can be caused by myocardial damage, hypoxia, increased sympathetic influence, or drugs.

Identifying Features

Rhythm: regular
Rate: 150–250 beats/minute
P wave: differs from sinus P wave, or may be lost in the T wave
PRI: .12–.20 seconds and constant
QRS: less than .12 seconds

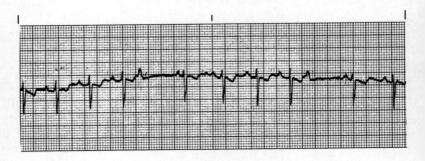

Clinical Picture

- rapid regular pulse
- patient is aware of increased heart rate and may exhibit signs or symptoms of decreased cardiac output or CHF
- atrial tachycardia is extremely dangerous in the presence of an MI because it increases myocardial oxygen consumption and workload

Treatment

This arrhythmia is usually converted by vagal stimulation such as Valsalva's maneuver or carotid sinus massage (CSM). If these maneuvers are unsuccessful, medications such as digitalis or Inderal may be useful in slowing ventricular response or converting the arrhythmia. In extreme cases, when the patient's cardiac output has dropped and the above methods of conversion have failed, synchronized cardioversion may become necessary.

Special Note

When atrial tachycardia is paroxysmal in nature, that is, it starts and stops very suddenly, it is called Paroxysmal Atrial Tachycardia (PAT). Treatment is usually unnecessary because it doesn't last long and converts spontaneously.

ATRIAL FLUTTER

Etiology

Atrial flutter is caused by an irritable focus within the atrium which initiates regular impulses at a rate of 250–350 beats per minute, thus causing the atria to contract at an extremely rapid rate. To prevent all of the impulses from reaching the ventricles, the AV node blocks some of them, thereby creating a ratio between P waves and QRS complexes, usually in a pattern of 2:1, 4:1, or 6:1. Sometimes this conduction ratio varies, causing the ventricular rhythm to be irregular. Atrial activity is represented by a sawtooth appearance, and ventricular conduction is normal.

Identifying Features

Rhythm:	atrial rhythm is regular; ventricular rhythm is usually regular but can be irregular if there is variable block
Rate:	atrial rate is 250–350 beats/min; ventricular rate varies
P wave:	called "flutter waves"; characteristic sawtooth pattern
PRI:	unable to measure
QRS:	less than .12 seconds

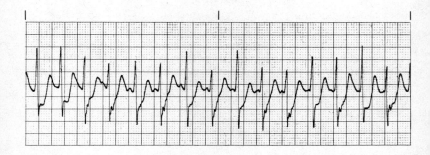

Clinical Picture

- can only be identified by EKG
- a rapid ventricular rate may cause the patient to complain of palpitations, angina, or dyspnea
- a rapid ventricular rate and loss of the atrial kick can cause decreased cardiac output or increased myocardial oxygen consumption, which can in turn cause CHF or myocardial ischemia

Treatment

Field treatment is necessary only if the patient has a fast ventricular rate with signs or symptoms of decreased cardiac output. Treatment is aimed at terminating the atrial flutter or slowing the ventricular rate by increasing the block at the AV node. Field management includes Inderal, Digoxin, and/or cardioversion. Carotid sinus massage or other vagotonic maneuvers may be tried, but usually slow the rate temporarily rather than converting the arrhythmia.

ATRIAL FIBRILLATION

Etiology

In atrial fibrillation, the atria become extremely irritable, and many ectopic foci initiate impulses at a very rapid rate. Because the atria are bombarded by multiple impulses, they are unable to contract and merely quiver ineffectively. Since the atria are twitching, the atrial pattern on the EKG shows fibrillatory waves but no discernable P waves. Due to the inability of the ventricles to accept these rapid-fire stimuli, most of the atrial impulses are blocked at the AV node. Those impulses that are conducted reach the ventricles randomly, thus producing an irregularly irregular ventricular rhythm, i.e., there is no pattern to the irregularity. Atrial fibrillation is usually distinguishable from other arrhythmias because it is *irregularly irregular* and has *no discernible P waves*. However, when atrial fibrillation becomes extremely rapid or extremely slow, the R–R irregularity might not be so obvious.

Identifying Features

Rhythm: irregularly irregular
Rate: atrial rate is greater than 350 beats/min; ventricular rate varies greatly (less than 100 is considered controlled, greater than 100 is uncontrolled)
P Wave: no discernible P waves; atrial activity is referred to as fibrillatory waves
PRI: unable to measure
QRS: less than .12 seconds

Clinical Picture

- irregular pulse
- patient may be aware of irregular heart beat or may complain of palpitations if ventricular rate is rapid
- may create a pulse deficit because the volume of blood ejected with each heart beat is not sufficient to produce consistent peripheral pulses
- may cause dyspnea or angina if the ventricular rate is rapid
- a rapid ventricular rate and loss of the atrial kick can cause decreased cardiac output or increased myocardial oxygen consumption which may in turn cause CHF or myocardial ischemia
- patients have a tendency to develop thrombi in the non-contracting atrial chambers, with subsequent threat of embolization

Atrial Fibrillation

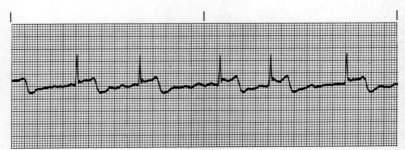

Atrial Fibrillation (Controlled)

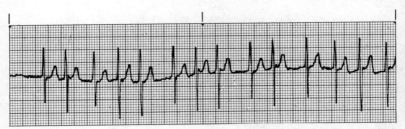

Atrial Fibrillation (Uncontrolled)

Treatment

This can be a chronic arrhythmia. Many older patients encountered in the field will be in atrial fibrillation and not require treatment. However, if the patient is showing signs or symptoms of decreased cardiac output due to a rapid ventricular rate, treatment should be instituted at once. As with atrial flutter, CSM and other vagotonic maneuvers are usually unsuccessful, necessitating the use of Digoxin, Inderal, or even cardioversion.

WANDERING PACEMAKER

Etiology

The SA node is the primary pacemaker in Wandering Pacemaker, but the site of impulse formation switches occasionally to the atrium or the junction. This may be caused by a speeding up of atrial or junctional impulses or by a slowing in the SA node. The shifting of pacemaker sites accounts for the variable P wave configuration. When the pacemaker site wanders toward or into the junction, the PRI may shorten and disappear. Conduction through the ventricles is normal.

Identifying Features

Rhythm:	normal or slightly irregular
Rate:	usually 60–100 beats/min
P wave:	morphology changes from beat to beat
PRI:	less than .20 seconds; may vary
QRS:	less than .12 seconds

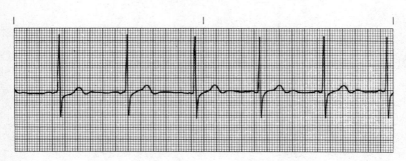

Clinical Picture

- does not cause symptoms
- identifiable only by EKG

Treatment

No specific treatment required. Watch for increasing incidence of junctional arrhythmias, as this may indicate myocardial irritability.

PREMATURE JUNCTIONAL CONTRACTION

Etiology

A premature junctional contraction (PJC) occurs when an irritable focus in the AV junction fires early and overrides the SA node. These ectopic beats can be distinguished from the sinus beats in Lead II because the P waves are inverted before or following the QRS complex, or are hidden in the QRS. The PRI is shortened and conduction through the ventricles is normal. An irritable junction may be caused by myocardial damage, hypoxia, or drugs.

Identifying Features

Rhythm:	underlying rhythm will be interrupted by early beat
Rate:	depends on underlying rhythm
P wave:	inverted before or after QRS, or hidden in QRS
PRI:	if P wave precedes QRS, PRI is less than .12 seconds
QRS:	less than .12 seconds

Clinical Picture

- irregular pulse
- patients are usually unaware of premature beats because they rarely produce symptoms
- identifiable only by EKG

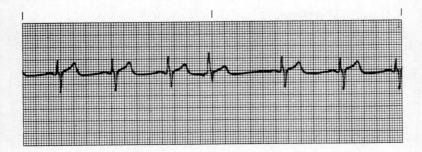

Treatment

Isolated PJCs are of little significance and can often be alleviated by oxygen alone. Watch the patient closely for an increasing number of PJCs or the onset of junctional arrhythmias, as this may be indicative of increasing myocardial damage and irritability.

JUNCTIONAL ESCAPE RHYTHM

Etiology

If the SA node becomes damaged or receives increased vagal stimulation, it may lose its pacemaker role. When the SA node slows, an impulse from the junction may then assume control and become the pacemaker of the heart. Junctional Escape Rhythm is a protective mechanism whereby the heart is able to continue to function despite failure of the SA node. As with all junctional arrhythmias, a single impulse is conducted in two directions. One flows retrograde to the atria; the other follows normal conduction through the ventricles. In Lead II, the retrograde conduction produces an inverted P wave, which may fall before, during, or after the QRS complex, depending on which chambers were depolarized first.

Identifying Features

Rhythm: regular
Rate: 40–60 beats/min

P wave: inverted; can fall before or after the ARS, or might be hidden in the QRS

PRI: if P wave precedes QRS, PRI is less than .12 seconds

QRS: less than .12 seconds

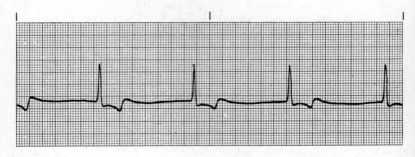

Clinical Picture

- slow, regular pulse
- can produce signs and symptoms of decreased cardiac output if rate slows significantly
- identifiable only by EKG
- may lead to heart blocks or ventricular standstill
- decreased cardiac output may occur and cause myocardial insufficiency
- may be an early sign of myocardial damage

Treatment

This arrhythmia is usually not treated unless slow ventricular rate causes signs or symptoms of decreased cardiac output, in which case atropine or Isuprel may be necessary.

JUNCTIONAL TACHYCARDIA

Etiology

In Junctional Tachycardia, an irritable focus in the AV junction speeds up and overrides the SA node, thus becoming the pacemaker of the heart. Junctional Tachycardia is an irritable arrhythmia, whereas a Junctional Escape Rhythm is protective. Atrial activity is represented by inverted P waves before or following the QRS complex, or hidden in the QRS complex. The PRI is shortened, but conduction through the ventricles is normal. Damage to the AV junction is the usual cause of this arrhythmia but drug overdose such as digitalis toxicity may also be responsible.

This arrhythmia is often subdivided by rate as either Accelerated Junctional Rhythm (60–100 beats/min) or Junctional Tachycardia (100–180 beats/min). Very rapid supraventricular arrhythmias often have indiscernible P waves, making a positive identification impossible. If P waves are not visible and the rate suggests several supraventricular arrhythmias, the rhythm can be loosely identified as a supraventricular tachycardia (SVT).

Identifying Features

Rhythm: regular
Rate: 60–180 beats/min
- 60–100 beats/min is called Accelerated Junctional Rhythm
- 100–180 beats/min is called junctional tachycardia

P wave: inverted before or after the QRS, or hidden in the QRS
PRI: if P wave precedes QRS, the PRI is less than .12 seconds
QRS: less than .12 seconds

Clinical Picture

- if the rate is fast enough it may produce palpitations or symptoms of decreased cardiac output
- identifiable only by EKG
- may progress to ventricular tachycardia or ventricular fibrillation
- usually indicative of advanced myocardial irritability

Treatment

If this arrhythmia is producing signs or symptoms of decreased cardiac

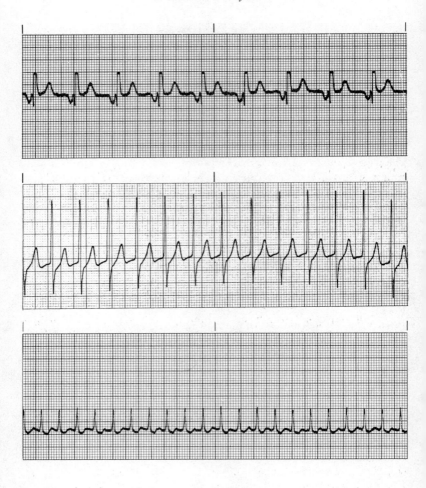

output, the irritable focus must be suppressed immediately. Junctional Tachycardia is usually converted by vagal stimulation such as Valsalva's maneuver or CSM. If these maneuvers are unsuccessful, medications such as Digoxin or Inderal may be useful in slowing ventricular response or converting the arrhythmia. In extreme cases, when the patient's cardiac output has dropped and the above methods of conversion have failed, synchronized cardioversion may be necessary.

FIRST DEGREE HEART BLOCK

Etiology

In the normal heart, impulses that arise in the SA node are delayed .12–.20 seconds at the AV node. In First Degree Heart Block, this delay is prolonged resulting in a PRI that is longer than normal but constant from one beat to the next. All impulses are then transmitted to the ventricles following normal ventricular conduction pathways. This arrhythmia may arise as a result of damage to the AV node, hypoxia, or drug overdose. You cannot completely identify an arrhythmia by calling it First Degree Heart Block alone. To be complete, the underlying arrhythmia must also be identified.

Identifying Features

Rhythm: depends on underlying arrhythmia
Rate: depends on underlying arrhythmia
P wave: normal and upright in Lead II; one P for each QRS
PRI: greater than .20 seconds; constant
QRS: less than .12 seconds

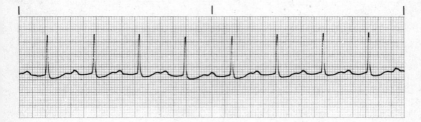

Clinical Picture

- patient is unaware of this arrhythmia
- no associated signs or symptoms
- can only be diagnosed by EKG
- not dangerous in itself but may forewarn of AV node injury which

could lead to more advanced heart blocks

- patient who has had syncopal episodes and is now in first degree heart block should be watched carefully for further block because he/she may be having Stokes-Adams attacks (episodes of intermittent 1st and 3rd degree heart block).

Treatment

First Degree Heart Block alone does not require field treatment, but it has the potential to progress to more lethal arrhythmias, or the underlying arrhythmia might be causing symptoms. Monitor the patient and transport to the hospital for follow-up care. Watch closely for increasing heart block, especially in the presence of digitalis toxicity, myocardial infarction, or recent syncopal episodes.

SECOND DEGREE HEART BLOCK MOBITZ I (WENCKEBACH)

Etiology

In Wenckebach, the SA node continues to initiate impulses in a normal fashion, but the AV node fails to conduct the impulses to the ventricles in a reliable manner. The delay of each impulse at the AV node increases progressively until one is blocked completely. This causes the PRI to lengthen progressively until one QRS is "dropped." Once the beat is dropped, the cycle may repeat itself in a regular pattern. This pattern is often referred to as "grouped beating." Ventricular conduction remains normal. Wenckebach may be caused by damage to the AV node, hypoxia, or drug overdose. It commonly occurs following an inferior MI and is considered relatively benign because the rate is usually adequate to maintain perfusion. However, it may progress to further heart block, so monitor patient closely.

Identifying Features

Rhythm: atrial rhythm is regular; ventricular rhythm is irregular; R–R interval becomes progressively shorter as PRI gets longer

243

Rate: atrial rate is normal; ventricular rate is usually normal but can be slow

P wave: normal and upright in Lead II; not every P wave has a QRS

PRI: normal or greater than .20 seconds; becomes progressively longer until a P wave is not conducted, resulting in a dropped QRS

QRS: less than .12 seconds

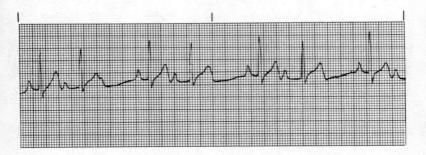

Clinical Picture

- patient may notice irregularity of pulse
- can only be diagnosed by EKG
- a sudden drop in rate might cause signs or symptoms of decreased cardiac output

Treatment

Usually does not require field treatment. Occasionally, the rate may drop and cause signs or symptoms of decreased cardiac output, at which point atropine can be very effective in increasing the heart rate. Watch for further heart block.

SECOND DEGREE HEART BLOCK MOBITZ II (CLASSICAL)

Etiology

In Mobitz II, the SA node is the pacemaker and every beat is conducted normally to the AV node. Upon reaching the AV node, however, only every second, third, or fourth impulse is conducted through to the ventricles. Thus, there is only one QRS complex for every two, three, or four P waves. On the impulses that are conducted, the PRI may be normal or prolonged, but it is *constant* with each conducted beat. The constant PRI is the key to diagnosing a Mobitz II. Conduction through the ventricles is normal. This arrhythmia may be caused by damage to the AV node, hypoxia, or drug overdose. Mobitz II is a dangerous arrhythmia because it may suddenly progress to third degree heart block or ventricular standstill.

Identifying Features

Rhythm: P–P interval is regular; R–R interval is usually regular, but can be irregular if block is variable

Rate: atrial rate is usually normal; ventricular rate is usually ½ to ⅓ that of the atrial rate

P wave: normal and upright in Lead II; more than one P wave for every QRS complex

PRI: may be normal or prolonged, but is *constant* on conducted beats

QRS: less than .12 seconds

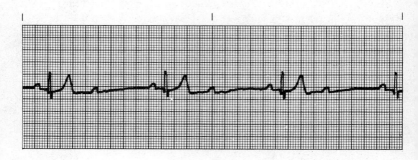

Clinical Picture

- patient may notice slow rate
- slow rate may cause signs or symptoms of decreased cardiac output
- can only be diagnosed by EKG

Treatment

Field treatment of Mobitz II is aimed at improving conduction through the AV node. If the patient shows signs or symptoms of decreased cardiac output, atropine may improve AV conduction and increase heart rate. If atropine is unsuccessful, Isuprel may be necessary.

THIRD DEGREE HEART BLOCK (COMPLETE HEART BLOCK)

Etiology

In Third Degree Heart Block, the SA node initiates impulses normally, but none of them is conducted through to the ventricles due to a complete block at the AV node. Therefore, the ventricles must be stimulated by either a junctional or ventricular escape focus, or ventricular standstill will result. The upright P waves indicate normal atrial activity, but the QRS complexes have no relationship to the P waves as demonstrated by totally inconsistent PRIs and an occasional P wave occurring in the midst of a QRS. The inconsistent PRI and the presence of AV dissociation are keys in differentiating Complete Heart Block from other heart blocks.

The QRS complexes may be normal or widened depending upon where the escape pacemaker originates. If the pacemaker is close to the junction, the rate will be 40–60 beats per minute and the QRS complex will be normal. If, however, the pacemaker arises lower in the bundle branches or Purkinje fibers, the rate will be 20–40 beats per minute and the QRS complex will be .12 seconds or greater.

Third Degree Heart Block is most commonly caused by damage to the AV node, but can also result from drug overdose. This arrhythmia is considered life-threatening because the rate frequently reduces cardiac output and may lead to asystole.

Identifying Features

Rhythm: P–P is regular; R–R is regular
Rate: atrial rate is usually normal; ventricular rate usually less than 40 beats/min, but may vary
P wave: normal and upright in Lead II; no relationship to QRS
PRI: characteristically inconsistent; no relationship between P waves and QRS complexes
QRS: less than .12 seconds if escape impulse originated in junction; .12 seconds or greater if escape impulse originated in ventricles

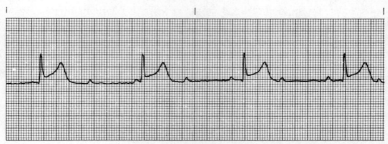

3rd-Degree Heart Block with a Junctional Escape Rhythm

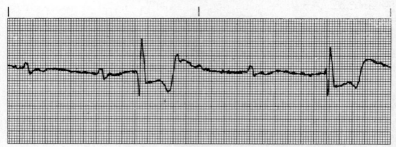

3rd-Degree Heart Block with a Ventricular Escape Rhythm

Clinical Picutre

- patient may show signs or symptoms of decreased cardiac output and may lose consciousness
- very slow heart rate
- this arrhythmia can cause Stokes-Adams attacks (transient syn-

copal episodes associated with intermittent periods of First and Third Degree Heart Block)

- patient may be in congestive heart failure

Treatment

Field treatment is aimed at increasing the ventricular rate to improve cardiac output. If the escape rhythm originates in the junction it will usually respond to atropine. However, if the impulse originates in the ventricle, Isuprel may become necessary. Field treatment is merely supportive; treatment of choice for this arrhythmia is the inhospital insertion of a pacemaker. Third Degree Heart Block may be temporary or permanent, depending on the extent of damage at the AV node.

PREMATURE VENTRICULAR CONTRACTIONS

Etiology

In a Premature Ventricular Contraction (PVC), an irritable focus within the ventricles initiates an impulse and overrides the normal pacemaker. The sinus node continues to fire but finds the ventricles refractory from the premature beat. Therefore, the P wave may be lost in the QRS or T wave. Due to the abnormal conduction through the ventricles, the QRS will be wide and bizarre (.12 seconds or greater). PVCs are usually followed by a fully compensatory pause unless retrograde conduction occurs, in which case the SA node can reset itself. Since PVCs are individual beats, the underlying arrhythmia must also be identified. The irritable focus within the ventricles may be caused by damage to the His-Purkinje system, hypoxia, acidosis, low potassium, congestive heart failure, or digitalis toxicity.

Identifying Features

Rhythm:	underlying rhythm will be interrupted by early beat
Rate:	depends on underlying rhythm
P wave:	usually lost in QRS; occasionally may be seen on the T wave
PRI:	none

QRS: .12 seconds or greater; wide and bizarre; T wave usually in opposite direction from QRS

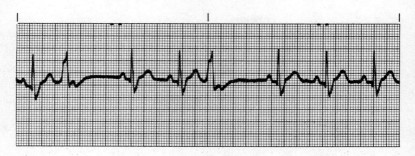

Clinical Picture

- most patients are aware of irregular beats
- an apical or radial pulse will reveal a long pause following premature beat

Treatment

Not all PVCs are considered dangerous. The following are circumstances in which treatment of PVCs should be considered:

- more than 5 PVCs per minute
- bigeminy, trigeminy, or quadrigeminy
- multifocal
- rapid succession of PVCs in a row
- "R on T" phenomenon
- any PVC in the presence of an MI

The aim of treatment is to suppress the irritable focus within the ventricles. Lidocaine works quickly to decrease ventricular ectopics. Oxygen should be used to correct PVCs associated with hypoxia.

VENTRICULAR TACHYCARDIA

Etiology

Ventricular Tachycardia (VT) is usually defined as three or more PVCs in a row. It may develop spontaneously, but usually is preceded by other signs of myocardial irritability such as PVCs. If P waves are present, they will have no relationship to the QRS complexes. More commonly, P waves are not visible because they are hidden in the QRS complexes. Ventricular Tachycardia is a form of AV dissociation, as the atria and ventricles beat independently of each other. Since the impulse arises outside of the normal conduction system, the QRS complex appears wide and bizarre and is .12 seconds or greater in duration. This arrhythmia is indicative of severe myocardial irritability and can advance very quickly to Ventricular Fibrillation.

Identifying Features

Rhythm: usually regular; may be *slightly* irregular
Rate: 150–250 beats/min; may be slower
P wave: may be present or absent; if present, has no relationship
            to QRS or is buried in QRS
PRI: none
QRS: wide and bizarre; .12 seconds or greater

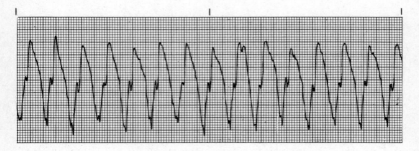

Clinical Picture

- if patient is conscious, will be aware of rapid heart rate

- can quickly develop signs or symptoms of decreased cardiac output
- cerebral anoxia may induce seizure
- peripheral pulses may be absent

Treatment

Because Ventricular Tachycardia causes a dramatic drop in cardiac output and progresses quickly to Ventricular Fibrillation, treatment must be initiated immediately. Field treatment is aimed at suppressing ventricular irritability. In a conscious patient, Lidocaine will usually convert the arrhythmia. In a patient who is unconscious or not perfusing, VT is best treated by cardioverting. Following conversion, Lidocaine should be given to prevent recurrence. Ventricular irritability in the presence of chest pain is very dangerous and should be treated immediately.

VENTRICULAR FIBRILLATION

Etiology

In Ventricular Fibrillation (VF), many irritable foci within the ventricles initiate pacemaker impulses, causing a rapid, repetitive series of chaotic fibrillatory waves. These waves have no uniformity and are bizarre in configuration. There are no identifiable P waves or QRS complexes, and the ventricles are completely ineffective as pumps. The exact mechanism that triggers Ventricular Fibrillation is unknown, but it is often preceded by a PVC falling on the T wave.

Identifying Features

Rhythm:
Rate:
P wave: grossly chaotic with
PRI: no discernible waves or complexes
QRS:

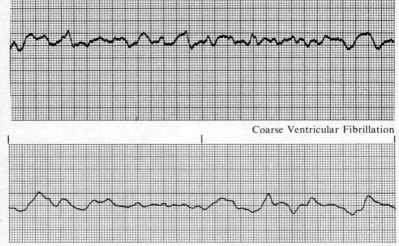

Coarse Ventricular Fibrillation

Fine Ventricular Fibrillation

Clinical Picture

- patient is unconscious and may seize due to cerebral anoxia
- patient is clinically dead; peripheral pulses, blood pressure, respirations, and heart sounds are unobtainable
- cyanosis and dilated pupils follow quickly

Treatment

Because poor electrode contact can create an EKG pattern very similar to VF, be sure to check patient's pulse before instituting treatment. Once assured that the patient is in VF, initiate CPR and continue BCLS for two minutes before attempting conversion. Then defibrillate and repeat once if necessary. Epinephrine and sodium bicarbonate can be given prior to a third defibrillation attempt. For frequent or recurring VF, consider lidocaine or bretylium. After conversion to a supraventricular rhythm, give lidocaine.

IDIOVENTRICULAR RHYTHM

Etiology

In Idioventricular Rhythm, the pacemaker function is taken over by the ventricles due to failure of both the SA node and the AV junction. This is the heart's final protective back-up system. The impulses are initiated at a rate of less than 40 beats per minute. Conduction through the ventricles is abnormal, causing a wider-than-normal QRS complex. Idioventricular Rhythm can follow any severe medical condition such as MI, drowning, or trauma. It is frequently the first arrhythmia found when assessing an arrested patient with paddle check. Idioventricular Rhythm commonly presents itself at some stage during most resuscitations. The electrical activity frequently fails to produce corresponding mechanical function or pulse (electromechanical dissociation). This arrhythmia is commonly described as being an agonal rhythm or dying heart.

Identifying Features

Rhythm: usually regular
Rate: less than 40 beats/min
P wave: none
PRI: unable to measure
QRS: wide and bizarre; .12 seconds or greater

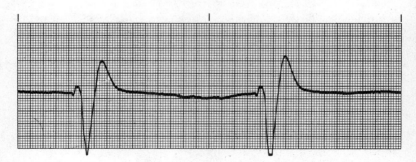

Clinical Picture

- if rate and perfusion are fairly good, patient may be awake, although sensorium will probably be altered

- if rate is low and perfusion is poor, the patient may have absent peripheral pulses, respirations, blood pressure, and heart sounds; patient is clinically dead

Treatment

This patient will probably require full resuscitation, and treatment should be instituted immediately. Therapy is aimed at enhancing higher pacemaker sites and increasing heart rate. Once sodium bicarbonate is on board, epinephrine, atropine, and/or Isuprel can be given. If mechanical function is also impaired, calcium chloride can be given to increase myocardial contractility. Lidocaine is contraindicated in this arrhythmia since it may result in asystole.

ASYSTOLE & VENTRICULAR STANDSTILL

Etiology

In *Asystole,* both the atria and the ventricles cease to contract because of absent or inadequate electrical stimulation. There are no P waves or QRS complexes on the EKG; only a straight line is visible. *Ventricular Standstill* differs from asystole in that atrial conduction may continue, but ventricular conduction is absent. This produces an EKG with P waves but no QRS complexes. Both arrhythmias are considered non-viable, and will result in death if not corrected immediately.

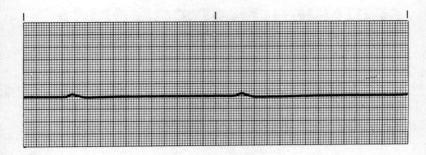

Identifying Features

Rhythm:	no ventricular activity
Rate:	no ventricular activity
P wave:	absent in asystole; present in ventricular standstill
PRI:	none
QRS:	none

Clinical Picture

- patient is unconscious
- patient may seize due to cerebral anoxia
- no obtainable pulse, blood pressure, respirations, or heart sounds; patient is clinically dead
- can only be distinguished from VF by EKG
- cyanosis and dilated pupils follow quickly

Treatment

Begin CPR immediately and start an IV. Give epinephrine and sodium bicarbonate IV push. If ineffective, administer calcium choride IV push. If rhythm is not restored, atropine may be administered. If Asystole persists, an IV infusion of Isuprel may be started, or epinephrine may be given IC.

FEATURES THAT COMPLICATE INTERPRETATION

ABERRANCY

Aberrancy refers to abnormal conduction through the ventricles. This occurs because one bundle branch is still refractory while the other is ready to receive a stimulus. This prolongs conduction through the ventricles and thereby causes a wide, bizarre QRS complex very similar in appearance to a ventricular complex. Aberrancy can affect a single beat or an entire rhythm. Aberrancy has no clinical significance and cannot be conclusively diagnosed in the field. To spend time trying to differentiate between aberrancy and a true ventricular arrhythmia can delay treatment and cause patient death. Therefore, when in doubt, assume the arrhythmia is ventricular unless you have legitimate reason to think otherwise.

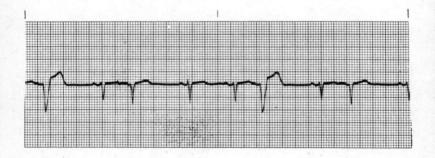

AV DISSOCIATION

AV dissociation is a term which is used to describe an arrhythmia, but is not an arrhythmia in itself. The term implies only that the atria and ventricles are functioning independently of each other. AV dissociation commonly occurs with Ventricular Tachycardia, Third Degree Heart Block, and PVCs.

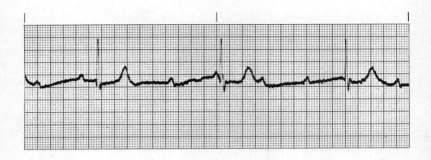

BUNDLE BRANCH BLOCK

This is not an arrhythmia, but a ventricular conduction defect that may be present in any arrhythmia. This phenomenon can be caused by tissue damage resulting from infarction or fibrotic scarring anywhere in the bundle branches. If only one bundle is blocked, the undamaged bundle conducts the impulses from the AV node to the Purkinje fibers of the ventricle it supplies. The impulse is finally conducted to the blocked ventricle by passing through the interventricular septum. The round-about path through the ventricles causes a wide, frequently notched QRS complex, usually .12 seconds or greater in duration. If both bundle branches become blocked, serious arrhythmias can result. Bundle branch block is difficult to identify positively on a single-lead rhythm strip. In the field, the patient's presenting signs and symptoms should guide management.

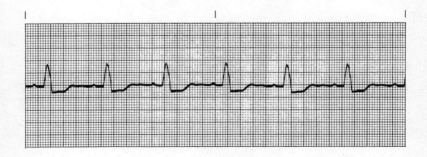

ELECTROMECHANICAL DISSOCIATION

Electromechanical dissociation is a condition wherein electrical activity is present in the heart but mechanical function is inadequate to sustain life. That is, the rhythm on the scope would be expected to produce a pulse, but the patient's pulse is not palpable. This condition can only be diagnosed by assessing the pulse while simultaneously looking at the EKG monitor. Electromechanical dissociation most commonly follows injury to the myocardium, as in cardiogenic shock or ventricular trauma. The patient is unconscious with no obtainable pulse or blood pressure. This patient requires full resuscitative measures with specific treatment aimed at improving myocardial contractility. The drug of choice for enhancing contractility of the heart muscle is calcium chloride.

ESCAPE MECHANISM

The heart has a built-in lifesaving mechanism that allows an impulse from the junction or the ventricle to escape and take over when higher pacing centers fail. This mechanism can take over for a single beat or for an entire rhythm. Escape beats can be differentiated from irritable premature contractions in that they come late in the cardiac cycle rather than early. Escape rhythms usually have a rate below 60 beats per minute. Escape beats and escape rhythms should not be suppressed; they should be supported. Atropine or Isuprel would be useful in enhancing higher pacemaker sites, but Lidocaine is contraindicated, as it would suppress the heart's failsafe mechanism.

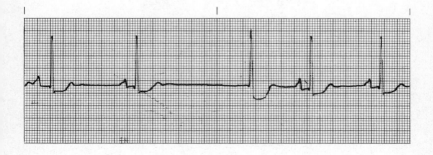

IRRITABILITY

When a pacing site within the atrium, junction, or ventricles suddenly speeds up and overrides higher pacemaker sites, it assumes pacemaking control over the heart. This process is called irritability. It can take over for a single beat or for an entire rhythm. Irritability is an undesired phenomenon, as it overrides the heart's normal pacemaker and causes an unusually fast rate. It can also progress to lethal arrhythmias if left untreated. Irritable beats can be distinguished from escape beats because an irritable contraction is premature, that is, it comes earlier than expected in the cardiac cycle. Escape beats, on the other hand, come later than expected. Treatment of irritability is aimed at suppressing the irritable focus. For supraventricular foci, vagotonic maneuvers, Digoxin or Inderal, and/or cardioversion may be tried. For ventricular irritability, Lidocaine is the drug of choice, in conjunction with cardioversion or defibrillation if necessary.

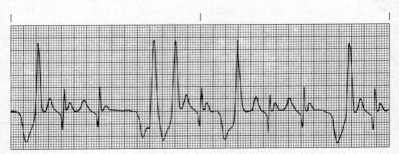

NON-CONDUCTED PACs

Occasionally, a premature atrial beat will occur that is not conducted through the ventricles because they are refractory. This is called a non-conducted, or blocked, PAC. The P wave has a different morphology than the sinus P waves, occurs early in the cardiac cycle, and is not followed by a QRS complex. This arrhythmia is often confused with Mobitz II (Wenckebach) but can be differentiated by measuring the P–P interval. In Mobitz II, the P–P interval is regular, whereas a rhythm with a blocked PAC will produce an irregular P–P interval. If these beats occur frequently they can cause a drop in cardiac output and might need to be treated with atropine.

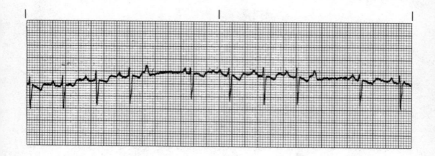

PACEMAKERS

If the electrical system of the heart fails, it is possible to stimulate the myocardium with an external source. An electrode pacing wire is placed in either the atrium or ventricle and connected to a pulse generator which discharges electrical impulses at a given rate. Because the electrode is in direct contact with the heart muscle, this impulse stimulates myocardial contraction. The electrical stimulus is represented on the EKG by a spike or blip. Atrial pacemakers produce a pacemaker spike preceding the P wave, which stimulates a QRS with normal conduction through the ventricles. Ventricular pacemakers produce a wide, bizarre QRS due to the initiation of the impulse below the Bundle of His. At first glance a ventricular pacemaker rhythm looks just like a slow VT, but the spikes preceding the QRS readily identify it. Ventricular pacemakers are used more commonly than atrial pacemakers because they bypass the AV junction, which is frequently damaged by an MI. Three types of pacemakers are commonly seen in emergency situations:

Transthoracic Pacemakers: In an emergency, a thin wire electrode can be passed through the chest wall to provide direct electrical stimulus to the myocardium. Once in place, a battery-powered pulse generator is attached and set at a rate sufficient to produce a viable rhythm. This type of pacemaker insertion is limited to extreme emergencies, and is seldom successful. As a result, it is seen only infrequently.

Transvenous Pacemakers: This is the most common method of pacemaker insertion. The pacing wire is inserted through a venous cutdown and threaded into the appropriate cardiac chamber. Fluoroscopy is usually used to guide the procedure. Once in place, the pacing wire is attached to an external pulse generator. This type of pacemaker is generally temporary; if needed, it can be replaced with a permanent pacemaker.

Permanent Pacemakers: Patients can be sent home with a pulse generator implanted in the subcutaneous tissue just below the skin. The electrode wires are attached to the endocardial or epicardial surface to provide the pacing stimulus. Internal pacemakers are usually visible as a round bulge below the clavicle or in the abdomen. Emergency personnel frequently encounter patients with permanent pacemakers when they malfunction, causing severe cardiac disturbances.

Most pacemakers have a "demand" function. This means that the pulse generator is designed to sense the heart's contractions and discharges only if the heart actually needs it. The EKG strip should show either a sinus beat, or in its absence, a complex preceded by a pacemaker blip. If the patient has a permanent pacemaker, as evidenced by a subcutaneous implant, but no pacemaker blips are visible, try another lead.

Malfunctioning pacemakers can be caused by displacement of the catheter tip, a low or dead battery, perforation of the ventricular wall by the pacing electrode, or exposure to an unshielded microwave oven. Malfunctioning pacemakers can be identified by the absence of blips in a patient with a pacemaker, or by blips without a resultant QRS complex. Pacemaker malfunction is a serious condition because it leaves the patient to rely on his/her underlying cardiac function, which is usually a severe bradycardia or heart block.

Pacemaker rhythms are only treated if they are malfunctioning. Very often, severe bradycardias may result with a subsequent drop in cardiac output. If this occurs, treat the underlying arrhythmia by stimulating the heart with atropine, Isuprel, and/or epinephrine, and transport quickly for medical evaluation.

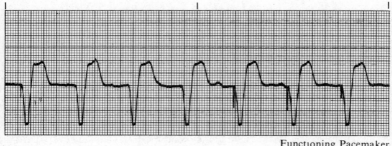

Functioning Pacemaker

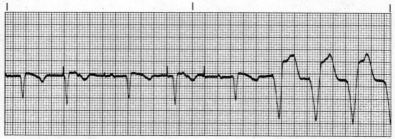

Malfunctioning Pacemaker

SINUS ARREST & SINUS BLOCK

In *SA arrest* the SA node fails to initiate an impulse at the expected time in the cardiac cycle. As a result, an entire PQRST complex is absent because no other pacemaker site takes over pacing. In *SA block,* the impulse is initiated normally but is blocked within the SA node and fails to reach the atria. Once again the entire PQRST complex is absent. These arrhythmias may be caused by damage to the SA node, increased vagal influence, hypoxia, or drug overdose, especially of Digoxin or Quinidine. If either of these arrhythmias persists, an escape beat may come in.

The patient is usually unaware of these missing beats, although a skipped beat may be noted. Palpation will reveal a prolonged pause with each missing beat. If the irregular beats occur frequently, cardiac output might be diminished, resulting in signs or symptoms of cerebral ischemia.

SA arrest and SA block are usually self-limiting and the patient does not require treatment. Occasionally, frequent or prolonged periods of SA arrest or SA block may produce signs or symptoms in the patient. If this occurs, atropine may be used to inhibit the vagal effect.

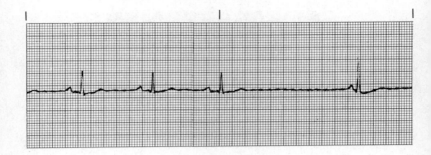

ST ELEVATION & ST DEPRESSION

Deviation of the ST segment above or below the isoelectric line may indicate myocardial insult as a result of coronary artery disease. *ST elevation* is consistent with injury associated with MI, pericarditis, or ventricular aneurysm. *ST depression* suggests myocardial ischemia, but can be a normal effect of digitalis. While ST changes seen on a field monitor aren't entirely reliable, they should not be ignored in patients with chest pain.

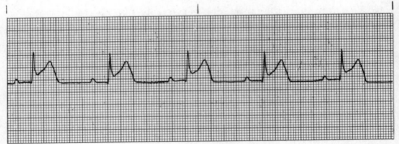

ST Elevation

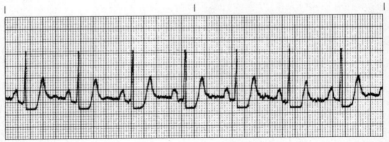

ST Depression

SELF-ASSESSMENT QUESTIONS

ELECTROCARDIOGRAPHY

FEATURES THAT COMPLICATE INTERPRETATION

14. How would you describe each of the following, including 2–3 distinguishing characteristics of each?

SELF-ASSESSMENT
SITUATIONS

1.

SITUATION: EKG of a 53-year-old male who states he has had the flu for several days and wants to go to the hospital. Vital signs are stable.

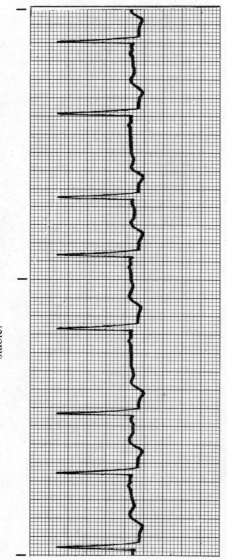

INTERPRETATION:

TREATMENT:

2. **SITUATION:** EKG of a 60-year-old male who has left sided weakness and difficulty speaking. Blood pressure is 160/110; respirations are 24 and regular.

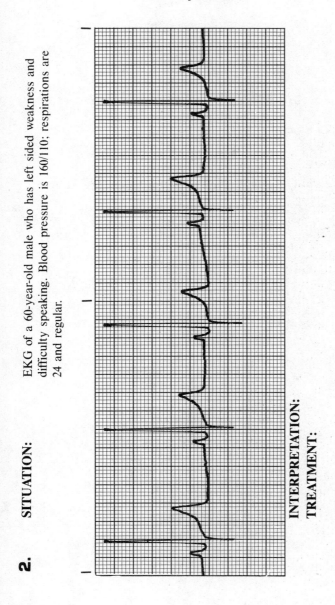

INTERPRETATION:

TREATMENT:

3. **SITUATION:**

EKG of a 62-year-old male who fainted and fell. He is now awake and alert and complaining of pain in his hip. Blood pressure is 110/70; respirations are 20; skin color is pale.

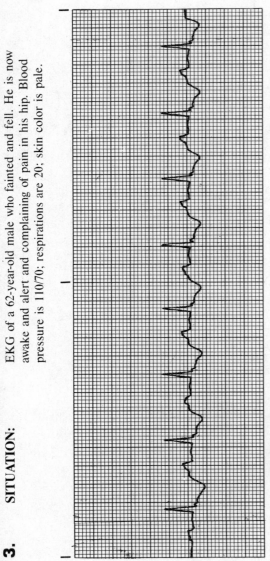

INTERPRETATION:

TREATMENT:

4. **SITUATION:** EKG of a 62-year-old female who was in a car accident and has a broken wrist. Vital signs are stable.

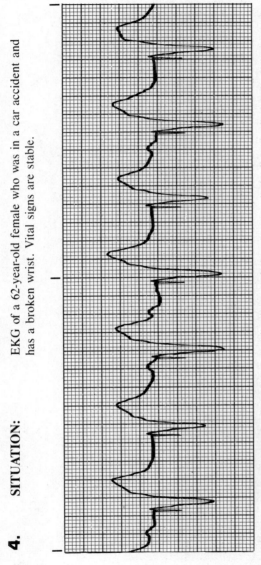

INTERPRETATION:

TREATMENT:

5. **SITUATION:**

EKG of a 46-year-old woman complaining of nausea, diaphoresis, indigestion, and shortness of breath. Her blood pressure is 126/92; respirations are 26. Skin is cool and pale.

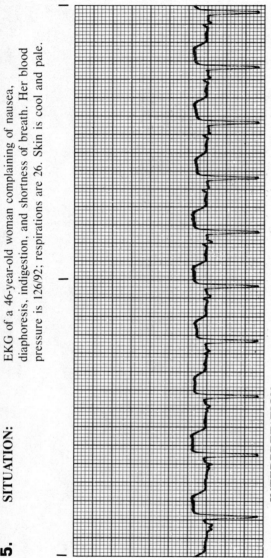

INTERPRETATION:
TREATMENT:

272

6. **SITUATION:** EKG of a 52-year-old male complaining of dizziness and palpitations. Blood pressure is 90/60. He is slightly diaphoretic and somewhat dyspneic. Lung sounds are clear bilaterally.

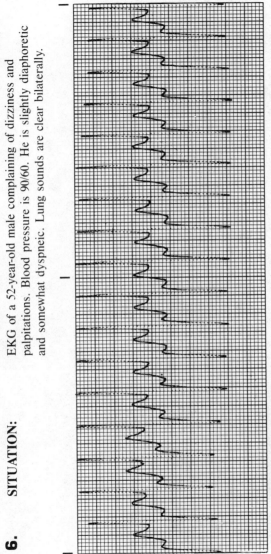

INTERPRETATION:

TREATMENT:

7. **SITUATION:** EKG of a 45-year-old male who experienced an MI one month ago. He is now complaining of pain on inspiration, hemoptysis, and severe dyspnea. Blood pressure is 120/90; respirations are 32 and shallow. Lung sounds are clear but diminished in the right upper lobe.

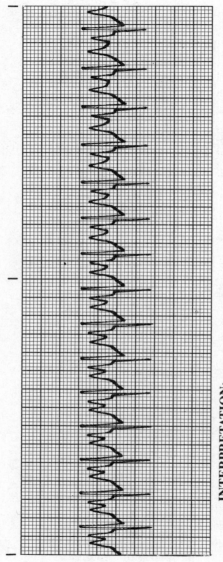

INTERPRETATION:

TREATMENT:

8. **SITUATION:** EKG of a 25-year-old female who has just been in a minor car accident. She has no apparent injuries and her vital signs are stable.

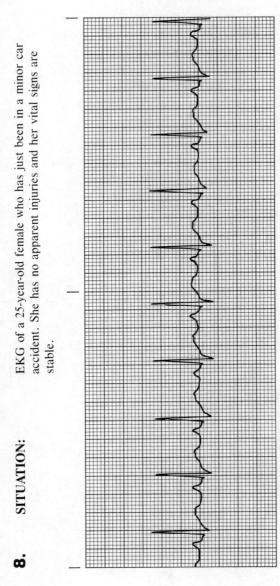

INTERPRETATION:

TREATMENT:

9.

SITUATION:

EKG of an 89-year-old female who was found unconscious by her housekeeper. She is now awake but disoriented. Her blood pressure is 90/60; respirations are 24; skin is pale and cool.

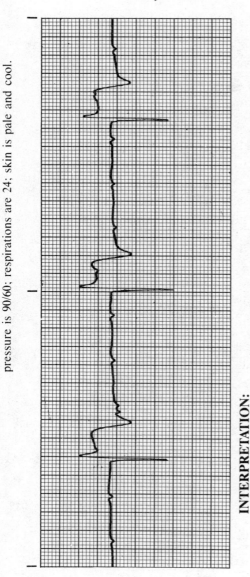

INTERPRETATION:

TREATMENT:

10. SITUATION: EKG of a patient who is becoming unresponsive and has no blood pressure or pulse.

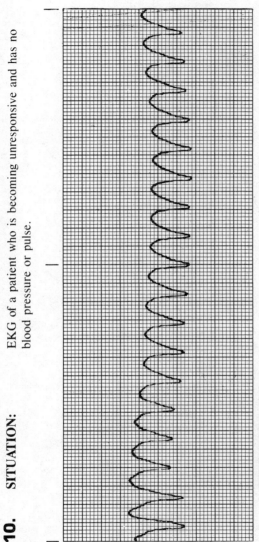

INTERPRETATION:

TREATMENT:

11. **SITUATION:**

EKG of a 45-year-old male complaining of severe, crushing, substernal chest pain of two hours duration. He is short of breath and nauseated. Blood pressure is 140/90; respirations are 28; skin is pale, cool, and clammy. Lung sounds are clear.

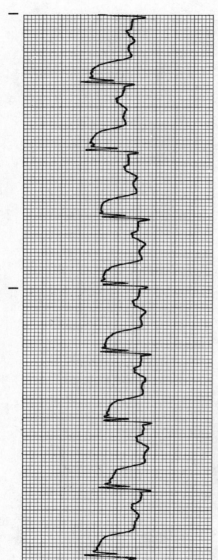

INTERPRETATION:

TREATMENT:

278

12. **SITUATION:**

EKG of a 30-year-old epileptic patient in a postictal state. His vital signs are stable.

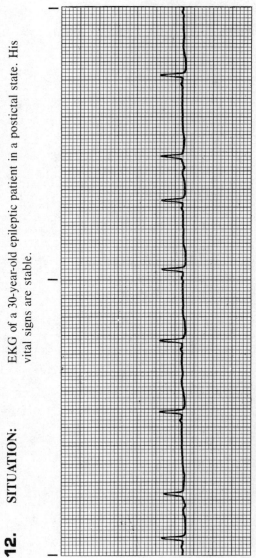

INTERPRETATION:
TREATMENT:

13. **SITUATION:** EKG of a 72-year-old patient with a history of heart disease who is on Digoxin orally. He is complaining of dizziness and has a palpable radial pulse of 30. His blood pressure is 90/70; respirations are 20, full and effective. His skin is cool, moist, and pale.

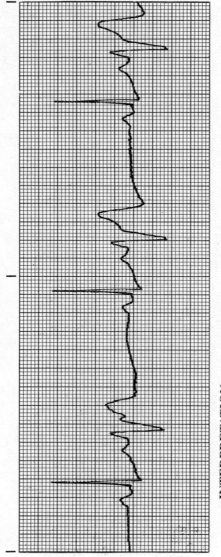

INTERPRETATION:

TREATMENT:

280

14. SITUATION:

EKG of a 45-year-old female who had thyroid surgery six weeks ago and is now complaining of pain in her incision line. Vital signs are stable.

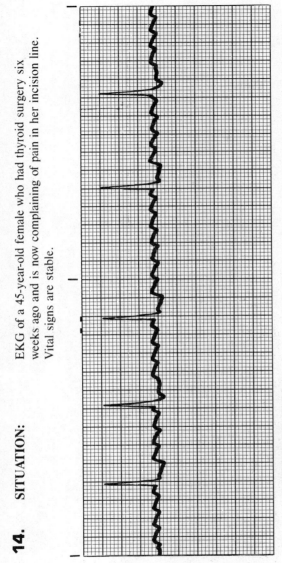

INTERPRETATION:

TREATMENT:

15. **SITUATION:**

EKG of a 23-year-old male who was just pulled from a swimming pool. He is unconscious, pulseless, and apneic.

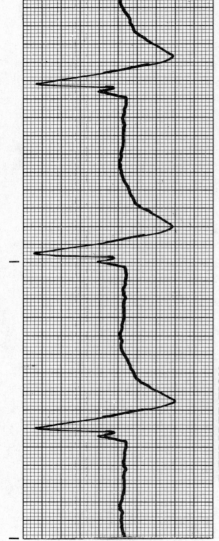

INTERPRETATION:

TREATMENT:

16. **SITUATION:**

EKG of a 53-year-old female who complains of gastric distress and says she has been vomiting dark coffee-ground material for two days. Blood pressure is 90/60; respirations are 24; skin is warm and dry.

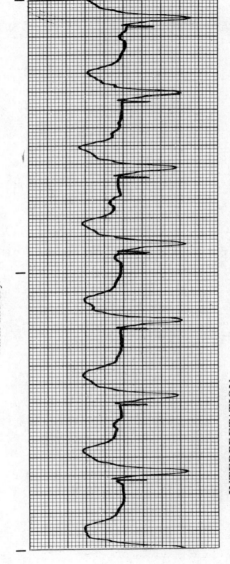

INTERPRETATION:

TREATMENT:

Arrhythmias

17. **SITUATION:**

EKG of an unconscious 27-year-old male, known to have overdosed on heroin. Blood pressure is 90/60; respirations are 8 and shallow.

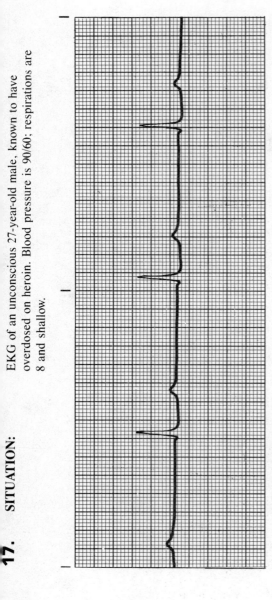

INTERPRETATION:
TREATMENT:

284

18. **SITUATION:** EKG of a patient who has just become unconscious, pulseless, and apneic.

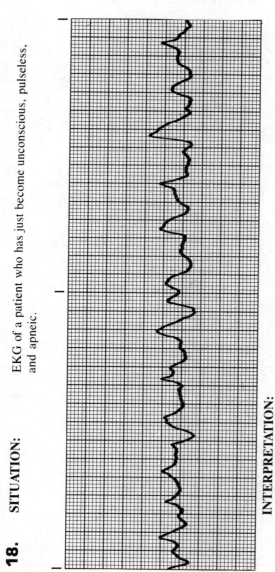

INTERPRETATION:
TREATMENT:

19. **SITUATION:**

EKG of a 65-year-old male who has had a pacemaker for two years. He is complaining of feeling dizzy. Blood pressure is 80/60; respirations are 18 and unlabored.

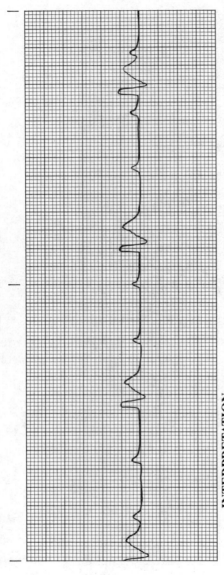

INTERPRETATION:

TREATMENT:

286

20. **SITUATION:**

EKG of a 51-year-old male with a past history of angina who is now complaining of chest pain after jogging. His pain has lasted 10–15 minutes. Blood pressure is 150/94; respirations are 24; skin is warm and moist. Lung sounds are clear.

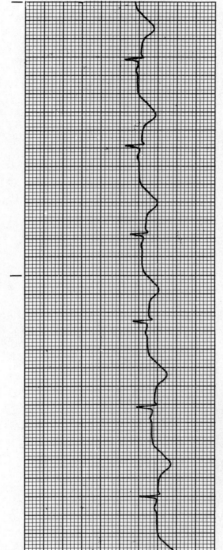

INTERPRETATION:
TREATMENT:

21. **SITUATION:**

EKG of a 45-year-old female who had valve surgery three years ago and is now complaining of palpitations and severe shortness of breath. Blood pressure is 140/90; respirations are 32 and labored. Lungs have rales and wheezes.

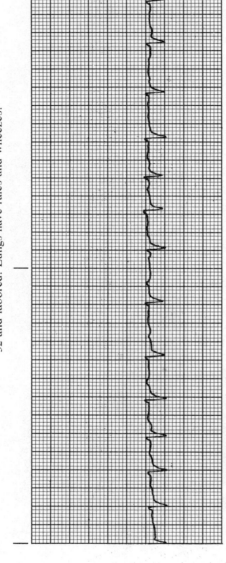

INTERPRETATION:
TREATMENT:

288

22.

SITUATION: EKG of a 29-year-old patient who was just stung by a bee and is complaining of severe respiratory difficulty. Blood pressure is 90/70; respirations are 36 and labored; skin is flushed, warm, and dry. Wheezes are heard bilaterally in the lungs.

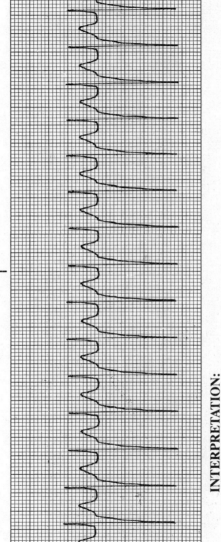

INTERPRETATION:

TREATMENT:

23. **SITUATION:**

EKG of a 19-year-old victim of a motorcycle accident. She has an open fracture of the femur with arterial bleeding. Blood pressure is 100/70; respirations are 24; skin is pale, cool, and clammy.

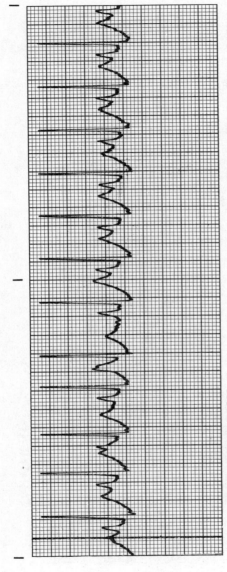

INTERPRETATION:

TREATMENT:

290

24. **SITUATION:**

EKG of a 62-year-old male who is experiencing severe heaviness in the chest. He has a history of atherosclerosis. Blood pressure is 110/70; respirations are 20, full, and bilaterally effective; skin is ashen, cool, and moist. Lungs are clear.

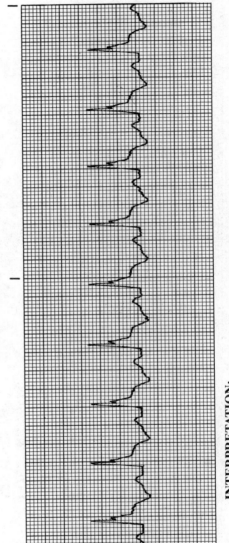

INTERPRETATION:
TREATMENT:

25. **SITUATION:**

EKG of a 55-year-old female who was in a car accident. Her only complaint is soreness across the precordium from where her chest hit the steering wheel. Her vital signs are stable; lungs are clear bilaterally.

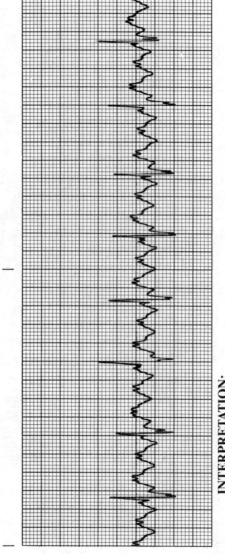

INTERPRETATION:
TREATMENT:

292

26. **SITUATION:**

EKG of a 28-year-old asthmatic patient complaining of severe dyspnea and exhibiting bilateral wheezes. Blood pressure is 110/74; respirations are 32 and labored.

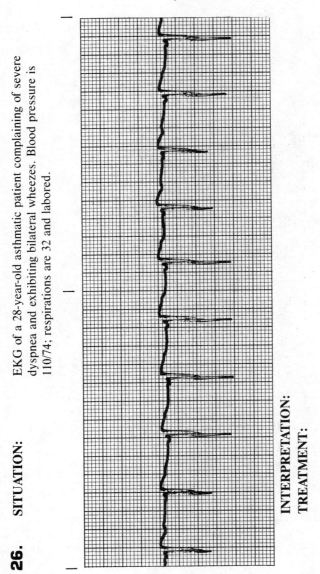

INTERPRETATION:

TREATMENT:

27. **SITUATION:**

EKG of a 46-year-old male who quit taking his Pronestyl at home and is now complaining of palpitations. Vital signs are stable.

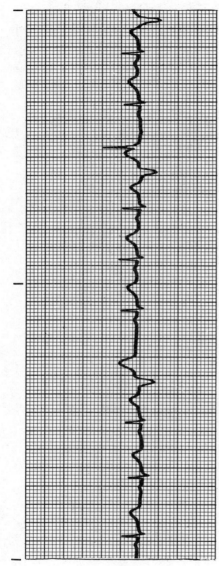

INTERPRETATION:

TREATMENT:

28. **SITUATION:** EKG of a 54-year-old female who presents with cool, clammy skin and decreased level of consciousness. Blood pressure is 80/54; respirations are 20; lung sounds are clear.

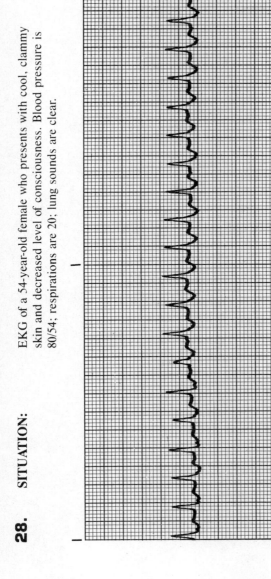

INTERPRETATION:

TREATMENT:

29. **SITUATION:**

EKG of an 85-year-old male awake and complaining of dizziness. Blood pressure is 92/66; respirations are 20; skin is pale, cool, and dry.

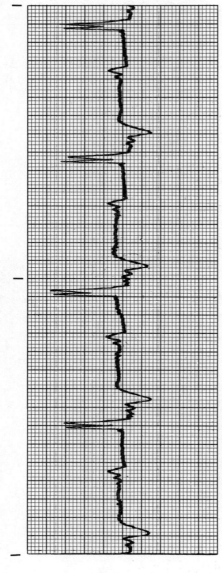

INTERPRETATION:
TREATMENT:

30. **SITUATION:**   EKG of a patient found unconscious in a rest home. He is now pulseless and apneic.

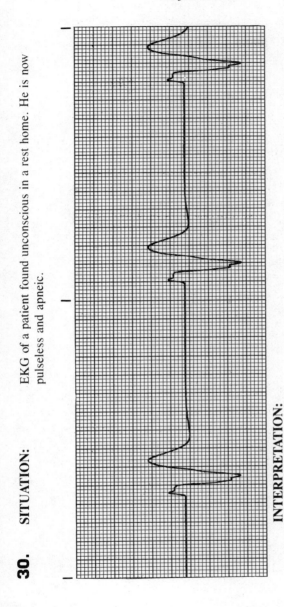

INTERPRETATION:
TREATMENT:

31. **SITUATION:** EKG of a 25-year-old male who was just pulled out of the ocean by a lifeguard. He is pulseless and apneic.

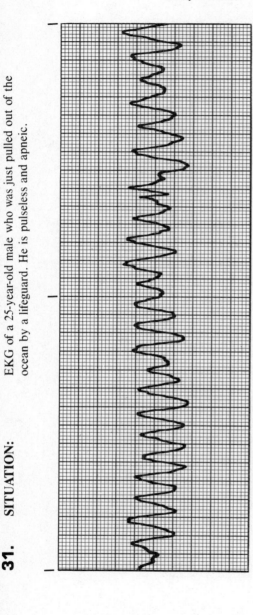

INTERPRETATION:
TREATMENT:

32. **SITUATION:** EKG of a patient who was bitten by a rattlesnake. He is complaining of pain at the site on his calf. Blood pressure is 130/84; respirations are 28 and shallow.

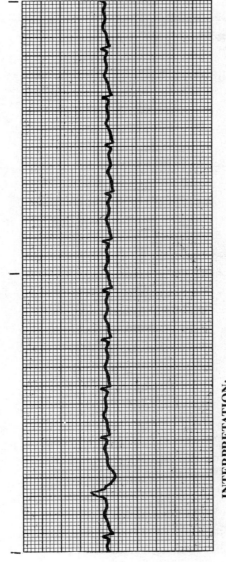

INTERPRETATION:
TREATMENT:

33. **SITUATION:** EKG of a 64-year-old male who has a history of heart disease. He is complaining of burning upon urination and colicky flank pain. Blood pressures is 122/78; respirations are 20 and regular.

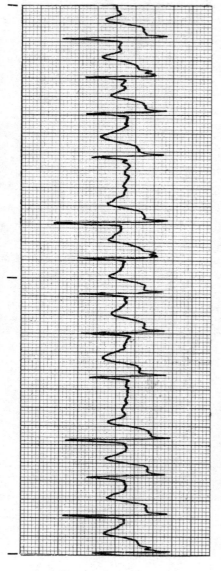

INTERPRETATION:
TREATMENT:

34. **SITUATION:**

EKG of a 34-year-old female with a history of psychiatric problems who is hysterical and complaining that she can't breathe. She has tingling in her fingertips and around her mouth. She has no history of heart or lung disease. Blood pressure is 128/78; respirations are 32 and shallow; lung sounds are clear.

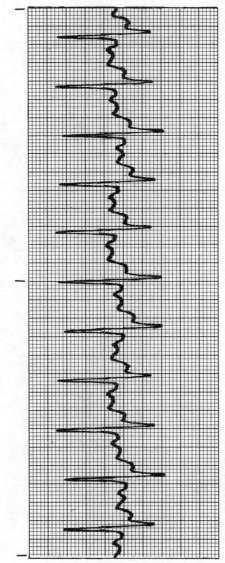

INTERPRETATION:
TREATMENT:

35. **SITUATION:**

EKG of a 28-year-old male working at an excavation site when a sandhill caved in, covering him completely. When pulled out, he was cyanotic. Blood pressure is 92/66; respirations are 10 and shallow. Lung sounds are clear.

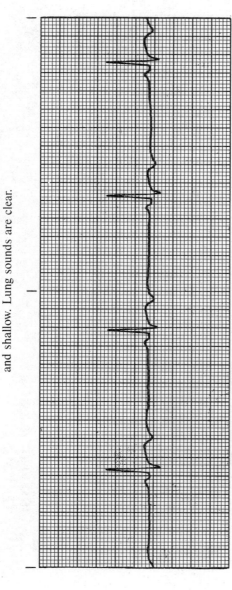

INTERPRETATION:

TREATMENT:

36. **SITUATION:** EKG of a 56-year-old male with chronic lung disease who is complaining of dyspnea. He is pale and diaphoretic. Blood pressure is 106/74; respirations are 32 and shallow. He has wheezes on expiration.

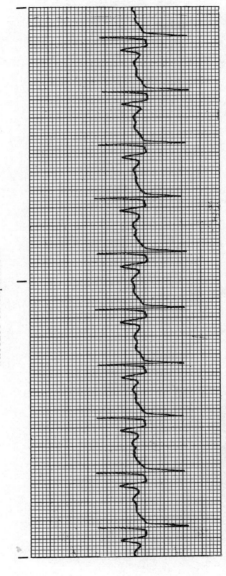

INTERPRETATION:

TREATMENT:

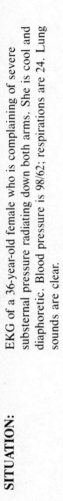

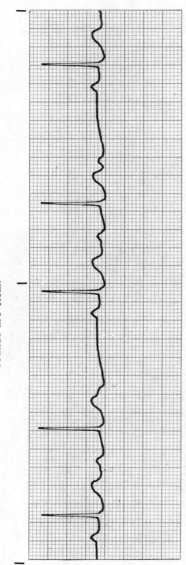

37. **SITUATION:**

EKG of a 36-year-old female who is complaining of severe substernal pressure radiating down both arms. She is cool and diaphoretic. Blood pressure is 98/62; respirations are 24. Lung sounds are clear.

INTERPRETATION:

TREATMENT:

38. **SITUATION:**

EKG of a 46-year-old male who developed chest pain while mowing his lawn. It has lasted for 30 minutes and has continued despite resting. He has no prior history of heart disease. Blood pressure is 140/94; respirations are 22. Lung sounds are clear.

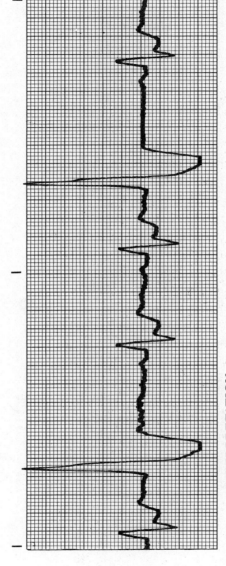

INTERPRETATION:
TREATMENT:

39. **SITUATION:**

EKG of a 3-year-old child who was trapped in an old refrigerator for two hours. She is conscious and crying, and color is good. Blood pressure is 92/62; respirations are 26 and unlabored. Lung sounds are clear.

INTERPRETATION:
TREATMENT:

306

40. **SITUATION:** EKG of a 42-year-old male who has just attempted suicide by taking 50 Valium tablets. He is conscious and has a strong gag reflex. His vital signs are stable.

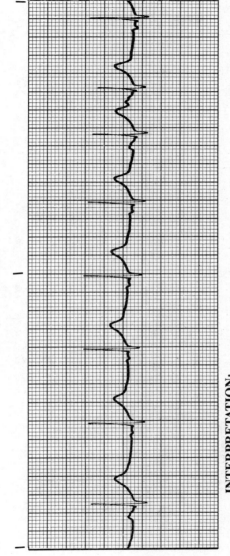

INTERPRETATION:
TREATMENT:

41. **SITUATION:**

EKG of a 65-year-old female who was awakened with a brief episode of shortness of breath and palpitations. She states that her symptoms are now returning. Blood pressure is 140/86; respirations are 30 and labored. Lung sounds are clear.

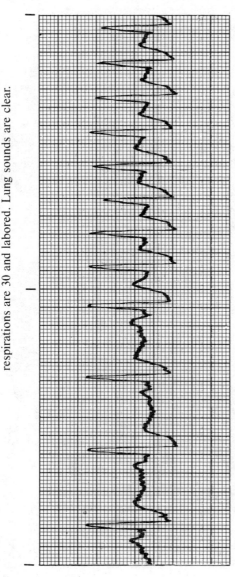

INTERPRETATION:

TREATMENT:

42. **SITUATION:** EKG of a 19-year-old male who has just been in a motorcycle accident and sustained a major head injury. There are no other apparent injuries. Blood pressure is 142/84; respirations are 12 and shallow.

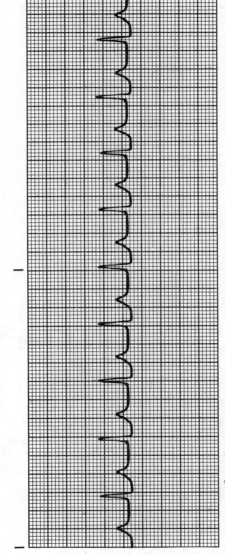

INTERPRETATION:

TREATMENT:

43. **SITUATION:** EKG of a 75-year-old who has a decreased level of consciousness. His blood pressure is 40/P; respirations are 28 and labored. Skin is pale, cool, and moist.

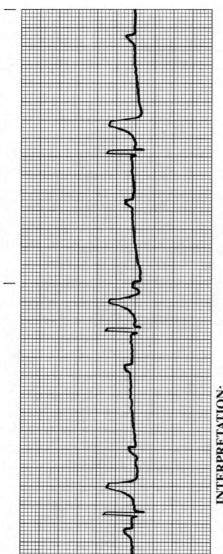

INTERPRETATION:

TREATMENT:

44. **SITUATION:**

EKG of a 52-year-old male complaining of severe, crushing, substernal chest pain with radiation down both arms, that has lasted for 30 minutes. He is diaphoretic, cool, and clammy. Blood pressure is 130/82; respirations are 24. Lung sounds are clear.

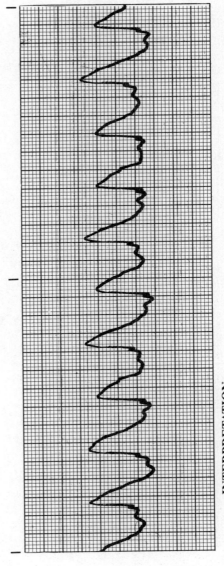

INTERPRETATION:
TREATMENT:

46.

SITUATION: EKG of an unconscious female who was found pulseless and apneic.

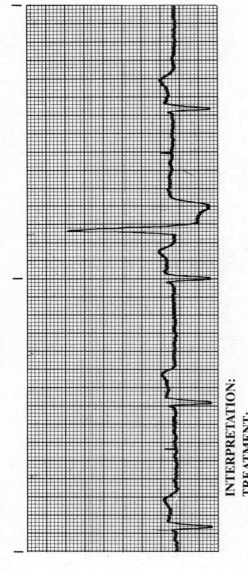

INTERPRETATION:
TREATMENT:

45. **SITUATION:** EKG of a 65-year-old female who collapsed in a restaurant. Blood pressure is 88/50; respirations are 26; skin is pale, cool, and clammy. Lung sounds are clear.

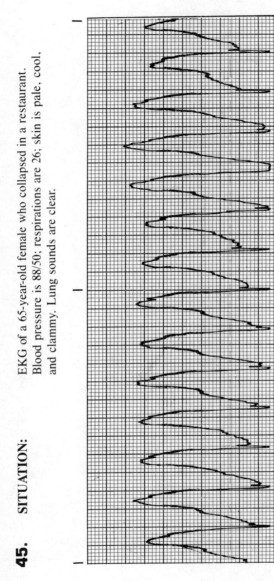

INTERPRETATION:

TREATMENT:

47. **SITUATION:**

EKG of a 53-year-old female just pulled out of a structure fire. She has sustained second and third degree burns to 45% of her body. She is alert, complaining of severe pain, and has no other injuries. Blood pressure is 136/80; respirations are 24. Lung sounds are clear.

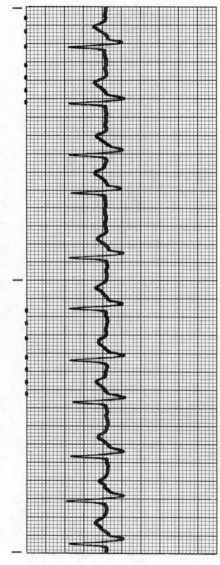

INTERPRETATION:

TREATMENT:

48. **SITUATION:** EKG of a 54-year-old male who was electrocuted in his home. He lost consciousness temporarily, but is now alert with stable vital signs.

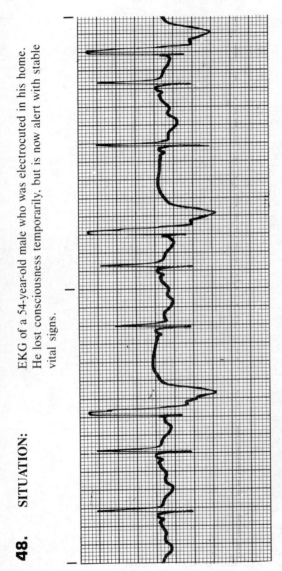

INTERPRETATION:
TREATMENT:

315

49. **SITUATION:** EKG of a 60-year-old female who is severely dyspneic and has a decreased level of consciousness. Blood pressure is 82/54; respirations are 32; skin is pale, cool, and moist. Lung sounds are clear.

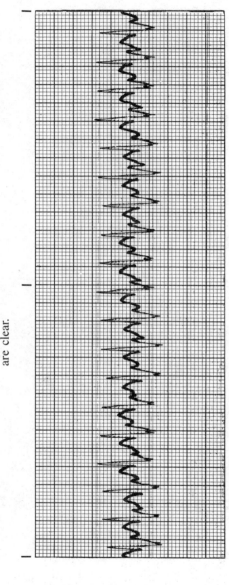

INTERPRETATION:
TREATMENT:

50. **SITUATION:** EKG of a 61-year-old male complaining of heaviness in his chest which has persisted for one hour. Blood pressure is 132/78; respirations are 16 and unlabored. Lung sounds are clear.

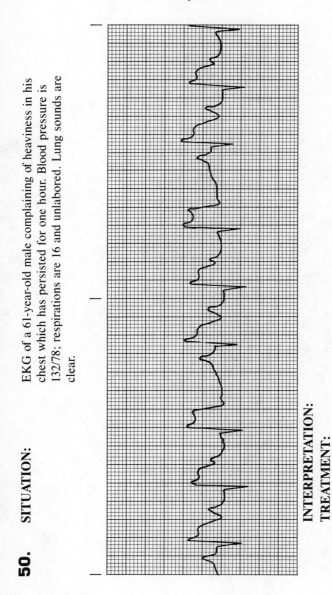

INTERPRETATION:
TREATMENT:

51. **SITUATION:**

EKG of a 73-year-old male who had complained of feeling light-headed and is now unconscious. Blood pressure is 94/64; respirations are 18 and regular.

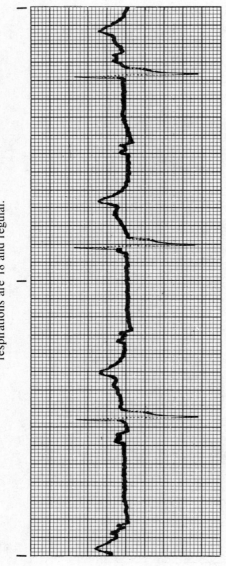

INTERPRETATION:

TREATMENT:

52. **SITUATION:** EKG of a 63-year-old female who has just been defibrillated for the second time.

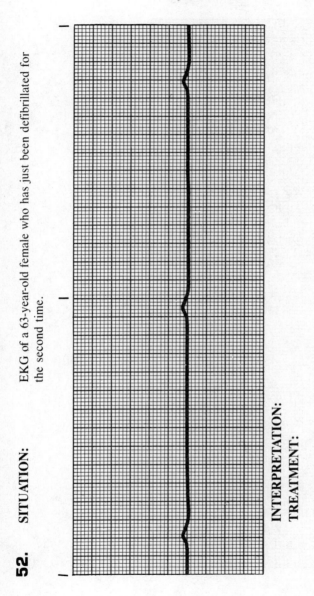

INTERPRETATION:
TREATMENT:

53. **SITUATION:**

EKG of a 20-year-old male involved in a hang-glider accident. He has obvious major head, chest, and abdominal injuries. He has no palpable pulse, blood pressure, or respirations.

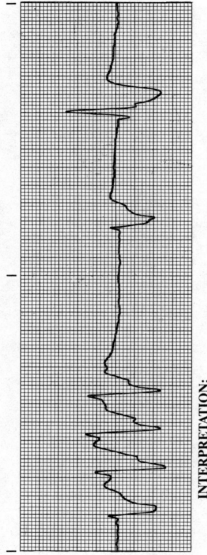

INTERPRETATION:

TREATMENT:

54. **SITUATION:**

EKG of a 56-year-old female who passed out while shopping. She is now conscious, coherent, and appears stable. Blood pressure is 138/80; respirations are 18.

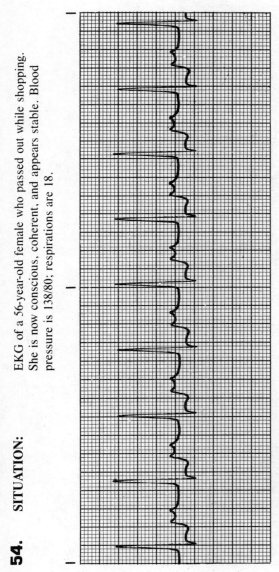

INTERPRETATION:
TREATMENT:

321

55. **SITUATION:**

EKG of a 14-year-old girl who was just pulled out of a swimming pool. She is breathing on her own but is unconscious. Blood pressure is 90/56; respirations are 14 and effective. Slight rales are heard in both bases.

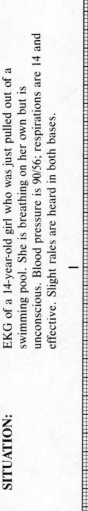

INTERPRETATION:
TREATMENT:

56. **SITUATION:**

EKG of a 58-year-old female with chronic lung disease who called you because she ran out of oxygen. Blood pressure is 152/94; respirations are 24 and slightly labored; skin is pale, warm, and moist. Wheezes are heard on expiration.

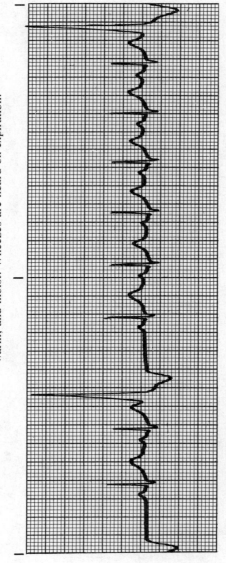

INTERPRETATION:

TREATMENT:

57. **SITUATION:**

EKG of a 54-year-old male who had an MI six months ago and is now complaining of crushing chest pain. Blood pressure is 124/80; respirations are 24; skin is cool and diaphoretic. Lung sounds are clear.

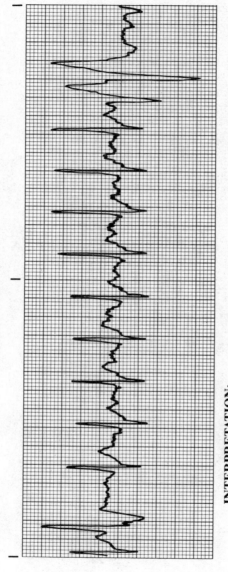

INTERPRETATION:
TREATMENT:

324

58. **SITUATION:**

EKG of a 72-year-old female in a physician's office complaining of substernal chest pain. The pain has persisted for the past two hours and has increased in intensity. She is slightly diaphoretic and anxious. Blood pressure is 138/76; respirations are 28. Lung sounds are clear.

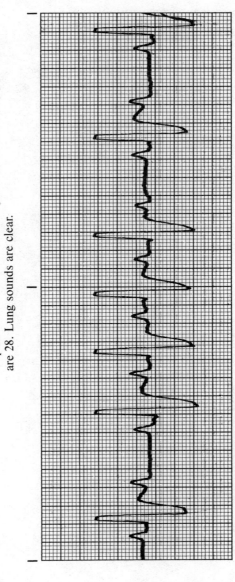

INTERPRETATION:
TREATMENT:

59. **SITUATION:**

EKG of an elderly man found unconscious, pulseless, and apneic on a golf course.

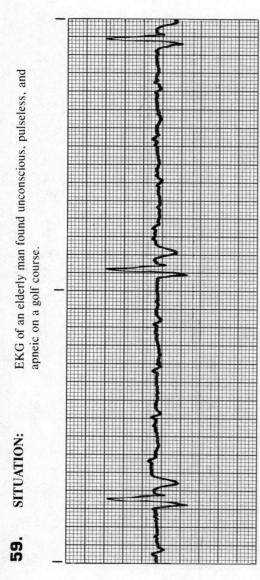

INTERPRETATION:

TREATMENT:

60. **SITUATION:** EKG of a man who reportedly doubled over suddenly with excruciating knife-like pain in his abdomen with radiation to his back. He then collapsed on the floor and is now pulseless and apneic.

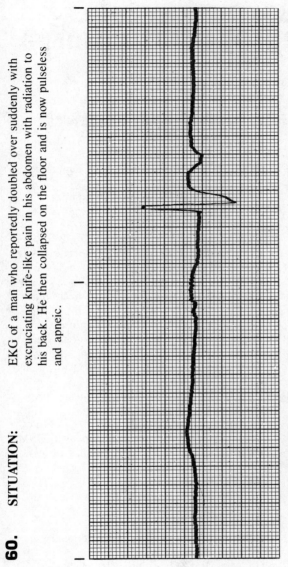

INTERPRETATION:

TREATMENT:

ANSWER KEY (SELF-ASSESSMENT SITUATIONS)

ANSWERS TO SELF-ASSESSMENT SITUATIONS

1. Interpretation: Sinus rhythm with 2 PACs, with depressed ST segment.
   Treatment: Oxygen. Watch for increase in number of PACs.
2. Interpretation: Sinus bradycardia.
   Treatment: Oxygen, IV TKO and consider $D_{50}W$.
3. Interpretation: Sinus rhythm with first degree heart block, depressed ST segment and inverted T wave.
   Treatment: Oxygen, IV (R/L or NS) TKO. Watch closely for progression into third degree heart block; stabilize the hip.
4. Interpretation: Pacemaker rhythm with good capture.
   Treatment: Splint wrist. Rhythm does not require treatment.
5. Interpretation: Wandering Pacemaker with deep Q waves and elevated ST segments.
   Treatment: Oxygen, IV TKO, morphine. Consider prophylactic lidocaine.
6. Interpretation: Supraventricular tachycardia.
   Treatment: Oxygen, IV TKO, Valsalva's maneuver, CSM, Inderal or Digoxin. Cardioversion if necessary.
7. Interpretation: Sinus tachycardia.
   Treatment: Oxygen, IV TKO, prompt transport.
8. Interpretation: Normal sinus rhythm.
   Treatment: No treatment necessary.
9. Interpretation: Complete heart block with a junctional escape rhythm.
   Treatment: Oxygen, IV TKO, atropine, Isuprel.
10. Interpretation: Ventricular tachycardia.
    Treatment: Begin CPR, cardiovert, IV TKO. After conversion, give lidocaine.

11. Interpretation: Sinus rhythm with elevated ST segment.
    Treatment: Oxygen; IV TKO; morphine; consider prophylactic lidocaine.
12. Interpretation: Sinus rhythm with 2 PJCs.
    Treatment: High-flow oxygen and IV TKO.
13. Interpretation: Sinus bradycardia with bigeminy of PVCs.
    Treatment: Oxygen; IV TKO; atropine. If PVCs persist after rate is increased, may need to treat with lidocaine.
14. Interpretation: Atrial flutter with variable response.
    Treatment: Oxygen, IV TKO.
15. Interpretation: Idioventricular rhythm.
    Treatment: Oxygen with positive pressure ventilation; CPR; sodium bicarbonate; atropine, Isuprel or Epinephrine; calcium chloride; nasogastric tube.
16. Interpretation: Paced rhythm with good capture.
    Treatment: Oxygen, IV (RL or NS), monitor vital signs closely.
17. Interpretation: Junctional escape rhythm.
    Treatment: Oxygen, assist ventilations; IV TKO, Narcan.
18. Interpretation: Ventricular fibrillation.
    Treatment: Precordial thump. Begin CPR. Defibrillate. IV TKO. After conversion give lidocaine.
19. Interpretation: CHB with ventricular escape focus.
    Treatment: O2; IV TKO; atropine or Isuprel; transport promptly for insertion of new pacemaker.
20. Interpretation: Sinus rhythm with depressed ST segment and inverted T wave.
    Treatment: Oxygen; IV TKO; NTG; morphine if no relief from NTG. Consider prophylactic lidocaine.
21. Interpretation: Atrial fibrillation (rapid ventricular response).
    Treatment: Oxygen; IV TKO; morphine, Lasix. Consider rotating tourniquets and/or Aminophylline.
22. Interpretation: Supraventricular tachycardia.
    Treatment: Oxygen; IV TKO. Epinephrine and Benadryl.
23. Interpretation: Sinus tachycardia with 2 PACs.
    Treatment: Oxygen; control the bleeding; IV (RL or NS). Bandage and splint fracture. Apply antishock trousers and be prepared to inflate.
24. Interpretation: Sinus rhythm with bundle branch block, elevated ST segment and inverted T wave.
    Treatment: Oxygen, IV TKO; morphine.

		Consider prophylactic lidocaine.
25.	Interpretation:	Atrial flutter (3:1).
	Treatment:	Oxygen, IV TKO, watch closely for EKG changes.
26.	Interpretation:	Junctional tachycardia.
	Treatment:	Oxygen; IV TKO; Isuprel or Metaprel Inhalant, epinephrine SC, and/or Aminophylline.
27.	Interpretation:	Sinus tachycardia with frequent unifocal PVCs.
	Treatment:	Oxygen; IV TKO; lidocaine.
28.	Interpretation:	Supraventricular tachycardia.
	Treatment:	Oxygen; IV TKO: Valsalva's maneuver; CSM; Inderal or Digoxin; cardioversion if necessary.
29.	Interpretation:	Second degree heart block (Mobitz II) with 2:1 conduction, bundle branch block, and inverted T wave.
	Treatment:	Oxygen, IV TKO; atropine.
30.	Interpretation:	Idioventricular rhythm.
	Treatment:	CPR; IV TKO, sodium bicarbonate, atropine, Isuprel, Epinephrine, calcium chloride.
31.	Interpretation:	Ventricular fibrillation.
	Treatment:	CPR defibrillate, IV TKO, Epinephrine, sodium bicarbonate, nasogastric tube.
32.	Interpretation:	Sinus tachycardia with one PVC.
	Treatment:	Oxygen, constricting band above the bite, cool packs around the site, lower the extremity and prevent movement, IV TKO, watch for increase in frequency of PVCs.
33.	Interpretation:	Atrial fibrillation.
	Treatment:	IV TKO.
34.	Interpretation:	Sinus tachycardia.
	Treatment:	Calm patient down, have her breathe into a paper bag.
35.	Interpretation:	Sinus bradycardia.
	Treatment:	Assist ventilations, IV TKO, consider Atropine.
36.	Interpretation:	Normal sinus rhythm.
	Treatment:	Low flow oxygen, IV TKO, Isuprel or Metaprel inhalant, Aminophylline.
37.	Interpretation:	Wenckebach (Mobitz I).
	Treatment:	Oxygen, IV TKO, morphine, consider Atropine.
38.	Interpretation:	Sinus rhythm with first degree heart block, bundle branch block and PVCs.

	Treatment:	Oxygen, IV TKO, lidocaine, morphine.
39.	Interpretation:	Sinus arrhythmia.
	Treatment:	Oxygen, IV TKO.
40.	Interpretation:	Wandering pacemaker with one PAC.
	Treatment:	Oxygen, Ipecac.
41.	Interpretation:	Sinus rhythm with bundle branch block, going into PAT.
	Treatment:	Oxygen, IV TKO, if PAT continues and patient develops a drop in cardiac output consider Valsalva's maneuver, CSM, Inderal or Digoxin, cardioversion.
42.	Interpretation:	Accelerated junctional rhythm.
	Treatment:	Hyperventilate, IV TKO, prompt transport.
43.	Interpretation:	CHB with junctional escape focus.
	Treatment:	IV TKO, atropine, or Isuprel. If BP does not increase with heart rate, give Dopamine.
44.	Interpretation:	Borderline sinus tachycardia with pronounced ST elevation.
	Treatment:	High flow oxygen, IV TKO, morphine. Consider prophylactic lidocaine.
45.	Interpretation:	Malfunctioning pacemaker with underlying junctional rhythm with a PVC.
	Treatment:	Oxygen, IV TKO, atropine, Isuprel, transport for insertion of a new pacemaker.
46.	Interpretation:	Ventricular tachycardia.
	Treatment:	CPR, cardiovert, IV TKO, sodium bicarbonate. After conversion give lidocaine.
47.	Interpretation:	Atrial fibrillation (rapid ventricular response).
	Treatment:	Oxygen, IV (RL or NS). Keep warm, cover burn, morphine as necessary.
48.	Interpretation:	Accelerated junctional rhythm with trigeminy of PVCs.
	Treatment:	Oxygen, IV TKO, lidocaine, check for associated injuries.
49.	Interpretation:	Supraventricular tachycardia (probably atrial flutter).
	Treatment:	Oxygen, IV TKO, Valsalva's maneuver, CSM, Digoxin or Inderal. Cardioversion if necessary.
50.	Interpretation:	Wenckebach (Mobitz I.)
	Treatment:	Oxygen, IV TKO, morphine, if rate slows consider atropine.
51.	Interpretation:	Complete heart block with a junctional escape rhythm.
	Treatment:	Oxygen, IV TKO, atropine, Isuprel, transport

for insertion of a pacemaker.

52. Interpretation: Ventricular standstill.
    Treatment: CPR, IV TKO, epinephrine and sodium bicarbonate, calcium chloride, atropine, Isuprel.

53. Interpretation: Agonal rhythm.
    Treatment: CPR, anti-shock trousers, IV (RL or NS), epinephrine and sodium bicarbonate, calcium chloride, atropine, Isuprel, prompt transport.

54. Interpretation: Sinus rhythm with first degree heart block with a depressed ST segment.
    Treatment: Oxygen, IV TKO, transport and watch for further block.

55. Interpretation: Wandering pacemaker.
    Treatment: Oxygen, IV TKO, consider nasogastric tube.

56. Interpretation: Sinus tachycardia with unifocal PVCs.
    Treatment: Low flow oxygen, IV TKO, consider lidocaine if PVCs persist. Consider Aminophylline.

57. Interpretation: Sinus tachycardia with multifocal and paired PVCs.
    Treatment: Oxygen, IV TKO, lidocaine, morphine.

58. Interpretation: Wencheback (Mobitz I).
    Treatment: Oxygen, IV TKO, morphine sulfate. If rate slows, consider atropine.

59. Interpretation: CHB with ventricular escape rhythm and underlying sinus tachycardia.
    Treatment: CPR, IV TKO, epinephrine, sodium bicarbonate, calcium chloride, atropine, Isuprel.

60. Interpretation: Agonal rhythm.
    Treatment: CPR, inflate antishock trousers, enroute start IV (RL or NS), epinephrine, sodium bicarbonate, calcium chloride, atropine, Isuprel.

SECTION IV: PRACTICAL SKILLS

CONTENTS: PRACTICAL SKILLS SECTION

INTRODUCTION

This section will help you review the skills used in providing advanced care in the prehospital setting. As with other parts of this book, the skills section was designed with the assumption that you already know how to perform these techniques; therefore, actual instruction is not included.

Twenty-seven commonly used skills have been selected and listed in alphabetical order. Each is summarized by a brief definition, along with indications, contraindications, and important points to remember when performing the skill. This short narrative is followed by procedural guidelines which list sequentially the steps that must be taken to complete the skill.

To use this section, you should first modify the procedural guidelines to comply with the teachings in your own area. Review the information provided and perform each skill under the supervision of your instructor or someone from your hospital. Then answer each of the self-assessment questions to ensure a total understanding of each skill.

Most of the skills included in this section were selected because they are used in many advanced life support programs in the United States. Some of the skills included are less widely used, but are considered vital by one or more specific training programs. Quite a few skills have been deliberately omitted from this review and may be noticed for their absence. All of the basic life support skills, e.g., cardiopulmonary resuscitation, bandaging, splinting, control of bleeding and extrication were excluded because they are covered in texts at the basic level. Several skills were omitted because they are impractical or they cause undue delay in the field, i.e., insertion of a urinary catheter and sophisticated auscultation techniques such as assessment of bowel sounds, fetal heart tones, and technical heart sounds.

Although most of the skills listed have fairly uniform performance criteria, some procedures must be modified according to the brand of product utilized in the performance of that skill. To facilitate explanation in these cases, specific brands were arbitrarily chosen for discussion. This does not imply endorsement of that brand. To modify such descriptions to fit the product used in your area, refer to your lecture notes, your instructor, or the product literature.

ANTISHOCK TROUSERS

Although several antishock trousers have been developed, each with individual identifying features, most consist of a basic three-chambered inflatable garment designed to cover the abdomen and lower extremities. The trousers are applied to hypovolemic patients to combat the shock state. The principles of action are: a) redirection of available blood from the lower extremities to vital organs, thereby increasing relative blood volume by about 1000 ml, and b) control of bleeding by direct pressure. The trousers should be applied as soon as possible following the injury and used in conjunction with other standard antishock measures.

The antishock trousers should be considered for any patient suspected of bleeding (internal or external) who is also exhibiting signs of shock such as diaphoresis, cool clammy skin, tachycardia, and a drop in blood pressure. Although most commonly used for hemorrhage following trauma, the antishock trousers have also been used in non-traumatic hypovolemic states, low resistance shock, and in cardiac arrest. Antishock trousers should be used cautiously in clinical states which are aggravated by increased intrathoracic or intracranial pressure. These relative contraindications include isolated head injuries, cardiopulmonary insufficiency, and major intrathoracic trauma. However, the trousers might be indicated in spite of the relative contraindication if profound hypotension is present and does not respond to other antishock measures. A strict contraindication for use of antishock trousers is pulmonary edema, since a sudden increase in blood return to the heart and lungs would further compromise the cardiopulmonary system.

The structure of the suit allows simultaneous or independent inflation of the three chambers. This flexibility allows the suit to be used in unusual circumstances such as pregnancy, bowel evisceration, marked abdominal distension, or presence of impaled objects. If an impaled object is present, it should be left in place and removed only as a last resort if all other treatment modalities are failing.

Apply the suit so that its upper edge is just below the rib cage and the lower edge leaves the feet uncovered. Make sure all Velcro straps are secure and all valves are tightly closed before disconnecting the inflated suit from the pump.

While the suit is inflated, monitor the patient's vital signs closely to avoid fluid overload. Watch for complications such as vomiting, aspiration, or difficult breathing. If any of these occur, deflate the abdominal compartment slightly to help relieve the pressure. Do not remove the antishock trousers suddenly, since to do so may throw the patient into sudden circulatory collapse and irreversible shock. Even in the hospital, the trousers should only be removed by a physician who is familiar with the garment, and then only when all support services are ready.

PROCEDURAL GUIDELINES

Three-Chambered Antishock Trousers; MAST III

1. Discuss indications for use of antishock trousers
2. Unfold garment completely and lay it flat on the ground or guerney
3. Attach foot pump and open stopcock valves
4. Place patient on the suit so that the top of the garment is just below the lowest rib and the feet are left uncovered
5. Wrap each leg of the garment around patient's legs and secure with Velcro fasteners
6. Position abdominal section and secure with Velcro fastener
7. Use the foot pump to inflate chamber(s) to about 104 mm Hg, or until air escapes through relief valves
8. Close all stopcock valves securely
9. Report to hospital that inflation is complete and provide an update on patient's condition

ASSESSMENT

Assessment of the total patient situation is the most important function you must perform. Without a systematic and thorough approach to assessment, vital aspects of the patient's condition might be overlooked. The order of assessment will vary according to each situation, but must always follow an organized format. Assessment techniques develop with practice but are rarely easy in the beginning. With practice and attention to detail, you can develop this skill into your most valuable tool.

The information presented here is offered only as a sample organized plan for all the information that must be remembered during patient assessment. It is vital that each paramedic develop his or her own organized approach, and use that approach consistently in dealing with patients in the field. For continuity, the entire assessment process should be completed by a single paramedic whenever possible.

The Primary Survey

Patient assessment is divided into primary and secondary surveys. The primary survey includes evaluation of the scene and initial assessment of the patient. First conduct a quick assessment of the scene to determine such things as a) the mechanism of injury, b) the number of patients to be treated, c) the need for extrication, and d) environmental dangers. During the primary survey, identify life-threatening situations and institute corrective measures. Your foremost consideration in all patients is the status of ABCs (see Table 1).

TABLE 1: ABC's

AIRWAY	• Is it patent?
	• Does the patient need positioning or suctioning?
	• Are the respirations noisy, gurgling, or labored?
	• Does the patient need an artificial airway?
	• Is the chest wall intact?
BREATHING	• Is the patient breathing spontaneously?
	• What is the rate, quality, and depth of respiration?
	• Does the patient need ventilatory assistance or support?
CIRCULATION	• Is the pulse palpable; if so, at which site(s)?
	• Does the circulation need to be supported?
	• What is the quality of the pulse?
	• What is the skin color?
	• Is there any obvious bleeding?

Each of these basic assessments must be made, and any deficiencies corrected, before continuing with a more sophisticated evaluation. During your primary survey you should also be looking for clues such as medication bottles, syringes, drugs or weapons. It may be helpful to request the assistance of auxiliary personnel to assist you in your survey of the scene; this also frees you for patient care.

After the ABCs have been assessed and necessary support given, you must quickly evaluate the patient and determine whether immediate transport is needed. There are circumstances which cannot be corrected by prehospital intervention because they require the sophisticated support available only within the hospital. These situations are generally those that require surgery, but can include any condition where prehospital intervention is not actively helping the patient. Examples of such conditions include dissecting or ruptured aneurysm, major trauma to the head, chest, or abdomen, or multisystem trauma, where the patient is not compensating or is deteriorating. Also if your system requires radio contact but your communications are disrupted, it is wise to transport the patient without delay, continuing assessment enroute.

The Secondary Survey

If the patient does not require immediate transport, move on to the secondary survey for a more detailed assessment. The secondary assessment consists of a) further investigation of level of consciousness, b) further investigation of the chief complaint, c) gathering of a pertinent medical history, d) assessment of vital signs, and e) performance of a manipulative physical exam.

Further Investigation of Level of Consciousness

If patient is alert and oriented without any suggestion of neurological impairment proceed directly to investigation of chief complaint. However, any patient with an altered level of consciousness or suspected neurological impairment needs more indepth assessment. The mnemonic BRIM can be a useful tool for this (Table 2).

Further Investigation of Chief Complaint

If the patient is conscious, determine why you were called and ask questions pertinent to the chief complaint. Pursue this line of questioning until a clear picture can be painted for the hospital. Avoid "tunnel vision" which can result from focusing on one problem before you have investigated other possibilities. The mnemonic "PQRST" can be used to guide investigation (Table 3).

The PQRST is a comprehensive approach to isolating the patient's problem. Once you have this information, specific questions can be asked to pursue your findings. For example, some specific questions to ask a patient who is having nontraumatic abdominal pain would include:

- Is there any change in the patient's bowel or bladder habits?
- Does the patient have any nausea or vomiting?
- Does the patient have any vaginal discharge?

TABLE 2:   BRIM

B	BREATHING	assess respiratory status	• What is the patient's respiratory rate, depth and effort? • Any abnormal respiratory patterns?
R	RESPONSE	assess level of consciousness	• Can the patient open eyes on command? • If so, is he oriented to person, place and time? • Does the patient respond to touch or deep pain? • If so, is the response appropriate, inappropriate, or neurologically abnormal?
I	EYES	assess eyes	• What is the pupillary size? • How do the pupils react to light? • Are the pupils equal? • What is the position of the eyes? Any deviation
M	MOTOR	assess muscle tone and movement	• Can the patient move all extremities on command? • What is the muscle tone of the extremities? • Are the hand grasps equal and normal in strength? • Is the strength of the legs equal and normal?

TABLE 3: PQRST

P	PROVOCATION	isolate precipitating or causative factor(s) associated with signs and symptoms	• What was the patient doing when the problem started? • Does anything make it better or worse?
		determine factors that aggravate or alleviate the problems	• Was there any trauma?
Q	QUALITY	patient's subjective description of the problem	• How does the patient describe the problem? • Is there pain? • Is it sharp, dull, aching, etc.? • Is there shortness of breath? • Is the patient having trouble getting air in? or out?
R	REGION	locate the area of involvement	• Can you point to the area with one finger?
		determine if the problem is localized or spreads to another area	• Does the problem stay in one area or does it radiate?
S	SEVERITY	determine intensity of the problem	• How severe is this problem? • How does this compare to previous similar problems?
T	TIME	determine chronology of events, including onset, duration and recurrence of symptoms	• When did the problem start? • Is it constant or intermittent?

GATHERING OF A PERTINENT MEDICAL HISTORY

A patient's medical history can often provide pertinent data regarding the present medical emergency. Some questions that may be asked to obtain the history may include:

- Is the patient taking any medications?
- What is the patient's past medical history?
- Does the patient have any allergies?

Gathering the Vital Signs

While obtaining a detailed history, begin to gather vital signs by palpating a pulse and assessing the quality of respirations. Other vital signs should be assessed as quickly as possible. Table 4 lists the factors to be determined and reported for each of the vital sign categories.

TABLE 4: Assessing Vital Signs

Vital sign	Factors to check
Blood pressure	systolic/diastolic; bilateral equality; response to position changes
Pulse	rate, rhythm, quality; response to position changes
Respirations	rate, rhythm, effort, effectiveness, patterns
Level of consciousness	response to stimuli (including voice, touch and pain); orientation;
Skin	color, temperature, moisture
Lungs	rales, wheezes, decreased or absent breath sounds
Pupils	position; equality; reaction to light
EKG	arrhythmias, correlation to pulse

Performing a Physical Examination

The data you gather from a physical examination should provide some clues to the patient's problem, as well as direct you to areas of further patient assessment. While obtaining the history and establishing the chief complaint, begin performing a rapid head-to-toe exam. A complete physical exam, with appropriate concentration on specific areas of complaint, can be done in less than 2 minutes.

Head-To-Toe Examination

Using the above assessment mechanisms, perform a rapid head-to-toe physical examination. Table 5 suggests a systematic approach that can be used.

When performing a physical examination, place emphasis on areas pertinent to the chief complaint. Some medical conditions, such as myocardial infarction (MI), may not require so thorough a manipulative examination as that indicated for trauma. However, an abbreviated but systematic head-to-toe review of the body will organize your evaluation of the patient and at least ensure that no other problems exist. In the abbreviated format used for specific medical complaints, some aspects of the physical exam can be omitted. For example, you may not need to palpate the neck for deformity and tenderness in an MI patient, but you should look for distended neck veins.

PEDIATRIC ASSESSMENT

Generally, the assessment of a child is the same as in an adult: perform a primary and secondary survey to include ABCs, chief complaint, vital signs, head-to-toe examination, special questions and a neurological exam when appropriate. However your approach in gathering this information should be different. It should be as gentle and nonthreatening as possible. Explain what you are going to do and what you expect from the child. In most cases, it is wise to have a parent present. You might leave a small child in the mother's arms, whereas older children may be asked to participate in their own care as the situation allows. An important point to remember when dealing with a child is to always be honest and straightforward.

TABLE 5:   Head-to-Toe Examination

HEAD	• Check for lacerations, hematomas, bleeding, depressions
FACE	• Check for cyanosis, pallor, flushing • Look for blood from ears, nose or mouth • Look for cerebrospinal fluid from nose, ears • Look for broken teeth • Note any obvious fracture of the jaw • Check eye movement • Look for diaphoresis
NECK	• Look at and palpate spine for tenderness, deformities, and rigidity • Check neck veins for distension • Check equality and quality of pulses • Look for tracheal indrawing and deviation
CHEST	• Look for paradoxical chest movement • Palpate thoracic cage for tenderness or deformity • Check accessory muscles for indrawing • Look for subcutaneous emphysema • Note scars from previous chest or heart surgery • Note barrel chest
BACK	• Note equality of chest movement • Look for bruises, injuries, entry or exit wounds • Check for sacral edema
ABDOMEN	• Look for bruises, penetrating injuries, distension • Palpate gently for rigidity
PELVIS	• Palpate pelvic girdle for tenderness or deformity • Note any urinary/fecal incontinence
EXTREMITIES	• Check pulses • Palpate all extremities for tenderness or deformity

- Check for strength of hand grasp, sensations, and movement of all extremities
- Check color and capillary refill
- Look for deformities, needle marks
- Check for pedal edema

Determining Pediatric Vital Signs

Vital signs will vary in the pediatric patient and you need to be familiar with these variations in order to be able to evaluate your assessment findings.

Pediatric vital signs vary from those of adults in that blood pressures are generally lower and pulses and respirations are generally higher. When taking a blood pressure on a child, be sure to use a pediatric cuff; the flush method may be used when auscultation is impractical. Table 6 approximates pediatric vital signs.

Body temperature in a child is also quite different from that of an adult, not in the actual reading but in the fact that it fluctuates so easily. This is why newborns are vulnerable to hypothermia and children frequently have febrile convulsions.

TABLE 6:   Vital Signs for Children

Age	Systolic B/P	Pulse	Respirations
Newborn	50	120	40–60
Child	70–90	95–110	20–30
10–15 years old	110–120	75–85	18–22

Estimating Pediatric Weights

Because pediatric drug dosages are calculated on the basis of body weight, it is important to remember general guidelines for estimating a child's weight in the field. The information in Table 7 refers to *average* children, and requires that you add or subtract weight depending on body build as well as age.

TABLE 7: Average Weight for Children by Age Group

Age	Weight
Newborn	7 pounds
6–12 months	15–22 pounds
2–9 years	add five pounds for each year
9–11 years	60–75 pounds

Reassessment

Assessment is an ongoing process. As field care progresses and patient condition changes, the assessment process should be repeated to monitor changes.

PROCEDURAL GUIDELINES

1. Conduct a primary survey
   a. evaluate scene, including environmental dangers, number of patients to be treated, need for extrication, mechanism of injury
   b. assess ABCs and correct any deficiencies
   c. collect data from scene, including medications, syringes, drugs, or weapons
   d. determine whether or not immediate transport is indicated
2. Conduct secondary survey
   a. investigate level of consciousness
   b. investigate chief complaint
   c. gather pertinent medical history
   d. assess vital signs
   e. perform manipulative physical examination, emphasizing areas pertinent to chief complaint
3. Modify assessment procedures to accommodate a pediatric patient
   a. recognize differences in normal vital sign values
   b. estimate weight according to age
   c. utilize family member(s) to facilitate exam process
4. Reassess patient as appropriate throughout run

AUSCULTATION OF CHEST SOUNDS

Chest auscultation is the act of listening to lung or heart sounds with a stethoscope. It is primarily used in the field to evaluate breath sounds and effectiveness of air exchange. Auscultation of lung sounds can detect rales, rhonchi, wheezes, absent and/or diminished breath sounds. It can be used in patients with respiratory symptoms, chest pain, unconsciousness, trauma or following treatment to assess effectiveness.

Since lung sounds cannot be adequately auscultated through clothing, place the diaphragm of the stethoscope directly against the patient's skin. As the patient inhales and exhales, listen to air exchange while systematically moving the stethoscope across the chest wall until all lung fields have been auscultated. Lung sounds are usually heard best from the posterior thoracic cage. Compare findings on the left side to those on the right side. Report the type of lung sounds and where they were heard.

During transport, reevaluate lung sounds, update vital signs, and report any changes in the patient's condition. This is especially important when medications such as Aminophylline or Lasix have been administered to alter the clinical condition. Chest auscultation is also used to evaluate heart sounds. Muffled or distant heart sounds, along with increasing signs of shock following trauma, should suggest pericardial tamponade. You might need to determine heart rate by auscultation. This is particularly useful in the presence of pulse deficit, or when no peripheral pulse is palpable. Detailed differentiation of heart sounds such as S_3, S_4, and friction rubs can delay transport and therefore should be reserved for hospital assessment.

PROCEDURAL GUIDELINES

1. Identify indications for auscultating the chest
2. Expose the patient's chest
3. Position patient
   a. have patient sit upright if alert
   b. if not alert, place patient first on back, then on side
4. Auscultate chest with diaphragm of stethoscope and check lung sounds
   a. instruct the patient to inhale and exhale through the mouth
   b. auscultate posterior and anterior lung fields in a systematic manner
   c. identify lung sounds detected
5. Place diaphragm of stethoscope over apex and auscultate heart sounds
   a. if respirations are noisy, instruct patient to

          hold his breath
  b. auscultate over apex of heart
  c. determine heart rate
  d. identify muffling, if present
6. Report findings

CARDIOVERSION

Cardioversion is the delivery of an electric shock to the heart by discharging a current directly to the chest wall. It differs from defibrillation in that the current is synchronized to be delivered on the QRS complex, thus avoiding discharge on the T wave. Cardioversion is used to convert uncompensated supraventricular or ventricular tachycardias. Supraventricular tachycardias are usually cardioverted in the field only after other techniques such as vagal maneuvers or drugs have been unsuccessful. Ventricular tachycardias should be cardioverted, rather than defibrillated, because they have T waves. Use caution when cardioverting a patient to whom digitalis has been administered, as this may result in ventricular fibrillation.

Start an IV TKO and sedate the patient with Valium if not already unconscious. Transmit the EKG throughout the procedure and give continuous oxygen.

Before cardioverting, be sure the synchronization button is on and that you can visualize the blip on the QRS complex. Select as low an initial watt/second (w/s) setting as possible for cardioversion of supraventricular tachycardia. Repeated attempts should be done at increasingly higher w/s settings. For ventricular tachycardia use the lowest w/s setting initially; if unsuccessful, use the full output of the defibrillator. As with defibrillation, use adequate paddle pressure and apply the appropriate amount of gel or saline. All other safety precautions are the same as with defibrillation. Following delivery of countershock, assess the patient for improvement in vital signs, level of consciousness, and rhythm. If necessary, repeat cardioversion at the same or increased w/s or resume other resuscitative measures such as CPR and drugs.

PROCEDURAL GUIDELINES	1. Identify the clinical indications for cardioversion in supraventricular and ventricular tachycardias
	2. Sedate the patient (if alert)
	3. Properly prepare paddles using gel, saline-soaked pads, or commercial pads
	4. Turn on defibrillator and select designated

w/s setting

5. Press Synchronization button and check for synchronization blip on QRS complex
6. Press Charge button and wait for full charge
7. Demonstrate paddle placement
   a. right: right sternal border, 2nd intercostal space
   b. left: at apex of heart
8. Apply paddles with approximately 15 pounds of pressure
9. Emphasize safety precautions
   a. wipe excess gel, saline, or perspiration off patient
   b. order "stand clear"
   c. keep hands off Discharge button until actually ready to initiate cardioversion
   d. disengage from physical contact with patient during discharge
10. Simulate cardioversion on a special manikin or replace paddles in unit and discharge current
11. Check EKG and vital signs to evaluate patient response
12. Discuss variations in technique for:
    a. anterior-posterior paddle placement
    b. pediatric paddles

COMMUNICATION EQUIPMENT OPERATION

Communication equipment operation refers to the use of radio hardware to establish two-way communication between the field and the hospital. Although communication systems vary greatly across the United States, most systems have basic components that are fairly uniform. In most areas of the country, the prehospital provider has at least two alternatives for field-to-hospital communication: the UHF mobile radio, and the land line telephone. Because of its flexibility, the portable mobile set is usually the first choice. If this frequency is crowded in your area, the telephone might be more appropriate if available. The ambulance-to-hospital frequency is usually reserved as a last resort when other methods are unavailable.

Ultrahigh Frequency Communications

All mobile radios used in the United States share the same eight frequencies allocated by the Federal Communications Commission for emergency medical communications. Because these frequencies are limited, the airways are extremely crowded in many high-density areas. In some areas, a central dispatcher selects an available channel for each call, while other areas rely on permanently assigned frequencies for each unit/hospital.

All of these mobile radio frequencies are ultrahigh frequency (UHF) and therefore operate "line-of-sight", i.e., any obstacle between the hospital and the scene (such as a hill or tall building) will interfere with and possibly prevent mobile radio communication. Sometimes communication can be improved by using a larger antenna or by placing the antenna on a large metal object such as a refrigerator or a metal vehicle. The major drawback to the field radio is the unreliability caused by "deadspot areas" where communication is poor.

To operate the mobile radio, first set the unit as close to the patient as possible. Then turn the unit on, select the appropriate channel and alert the hospital. In some cases this is done automatically with the first transmission, but in others it is necessary to send a few seconds of EKG calibration in order to alert the hospital that a run is in progress. When speaking, leave the radio in the push-to-talk mode, and turn to the calibration or EKG modes only for these purposes. If possible, leave the radio in the "mute" position to avoid broadcasting the hospital's transmissions to all of the people at the scene. All mobile radios have knobs for adjusting volume and outside interference. Leave the radio frequency open throughout the run so the hospital can contact you if necessary.

Telephone Land Lines

If a telephone is near the patient, it can be used to augment or replace mobile radio communications. This mode is often useful when frequencies are crowded, but is limited because telephones are not always available. Telephone conversations, like radio conversations, can be recorded at the hospital for documentation. The telephone can be attached to the radio's telephone coupler to enable the transmission of EKG telemetry to the hospital if desired. Use care in placing a Princess or Trimline style handset into the coupler, as they don't fit snugly and can be easily disconnected.

PROCEDURAL **Mobile Radio**
GUIDELINES   1. Open radio, select channel, and set up

antenna
a. small gain
b. high gain (if needed)
c. augment antenna (if needed)
2. Turn on radio to Voice or "Push to Talk"
3. Adjust volume and/or squelch as needed
4. Send short calibration signal to alert hospital (if needed)
5. Report patient data using an organized format
6. Mute speaker (if requested)
7. Send EKG signal (if requested)

Telephone Coupler
1. Contact hospital over direct land line
2. Attach telephone coupler and communicate through mobile radio over land lines
a. attach telephone coupler plug into radio
b. place phone handset into coupler and secure it
c. select proper radio mode
3. Transmit telemetry over land line via telephone coupler

COMMUNICATION FORMAT

Communication by mobile radio is a major component of advanced life support systems. It allows the exchange of pertinent information between the scene and the hospital, thereby facilitating management of medical emergencies before arrival at the emergency department.

The key to effective communication with the hospital is the use of an organized format for reporting patient information in clear, concise terms. By giving the hospital a rapid synopsis of the situation, you can help the hospital direct patient care more efficiently. In your initial report give a brief summary of the chief complaint, general patient status/severity and level of consciousness, as well as an overview of the scene. Avoid diagnosing the patient in your initial transmission, as this may mislead the hospital by limiting the information available to them. Follow this report with an organized summary of the data you have gathered about the patient including age, weight, and sex, a description of the present medical problem, pertinent history, physical exam findings and vital signs. Keep your reports brief and to the point. Use descriptive but appropriate terms, and convey your impressions to the hospital in addition to your actual findings. The specific situation and patient condition may require a varied report format, but always organize your thoughts and communicate them accurately. You might find it helpful to use the field report form as a guide for communicating.

Avoid unnecessary transmissions, as this will prevent you from assisting your partner and may interrupt the communications of other ALS teams. To prevent confusion among teams, identify your unit and your hospital with each transmission. In multiple patient incidents, report the most critical patients first, clearly identifying each by an assigned number.

Keep the hospital informed of your actions, particularly if the situation requires pauses in communication. Inform them of changes in patient condition as well as response to treatment. Always speak in a clear voice, maintain a professional manner, and use appropriate medical terms. Repeat all orders for verification, and be courteous and tactful if questions arise. Handle communication difficulties discretely, using alternate communication modes as needed.

If it is not possible to contact the hospital, and your area requires voice contact in order for you to perform advanced prehospital care, you should administer basic life support only and transport the patient immediately.

PROCEDURAL
GUIDELINES

1. Establish communication
   a. turn radio on
   b. select proper channel
   c. call hospital
   d. identify unit
   e. ask if hospital is copying transmission
2. Use good radio techniques
   a. volume, enunciation, and speed as appropriate
   b. use proper terminology
   c. be concise and express appropriate urgency
3. Give initial report (vary report according to urgency) and include
   a. overview of scene
   b. chief complaint
   c. patient status/severity
   d. level of consciousness
4. Report additional patient information
   a. age, sex, weight
   b. presenting medical problem
   c. pertinent history
   d. physical findings

e. vital signs
5. Acknowledge orders from hospital
    a. repeat exactly as heard and write them down
    b. question unclear orders
    c. provide additional data as requested
6. Report completion of orders and patient response
7. Sign off with final patient report and estimated time of arrival at the hospital

CRICOTHYROTOMY

Cricothyrotomy is the creation of an artificial airway in the trachea to bypass the site of an upper airway obstruction. It is a life-saving measure that should be performed *only* when all other methods of opening and maintaining a patent airway have failed.

The cricothyroid membrane is used because 1) it is easily located, 2) it can be quickly penetrated in an emergency situation, 3) it contains no vital structures, and 4) it is located below the vocal cords.

Bleeding is the most common complication of this procedure, but it is usually minor and controllable. Other complications include speech or nerve impairment (if the incision is made incorrectly), infection, or collapse of the cricoid cartilage itself. When performing this procedure, it is important to properly identify the landmarks and keep the incision small and in the midline.

Although the incision method provides greater air exchange, the puncture method is recommended because it is simpler and has a lesser potential for complications. To provide adequate air exchange, you may need to place additional cannulas adjacent to the first. After opening the airway, provide ventilatory assistance with high-flow oxygen. Following the procedure, transport promptly and monitor the patient closely.

PROCEDURAL GUIDELINES

Incision Method
1. Recognize indications for procedure
2. Select equipment
3. Place a small roll under patient's shoulders to slightly extend the neck
4. Locate cricothyroid membrane between the thyroid cartilage and the cricoid cartilage
5. Prepare the skin with antiseptic swab and maintain aseptic technique

6. Stabilize thyroid cartilage between thumb and middle finger of one hand
7. Press index finger of same hand between the thyroid and cricoid cartilage to identify the cricothyroid membrane
8. Using index finger as a guide, make a small scalpel incision (2 cm) through the skin at the midline
9. Make second incision through the cricothyroid membrane, taking care not to incise laterally or too deeply
10. Rotate knife handle 90° to widen opening
11. Insert a cannula, tubing, or penshaft to maintain an airway
12. Check placement of the airway by
    a. ventilating (as necessary) and watching the chest rise
    b. listening for air exchange at the site
    c. observing patient for color and respiratory improvement
13. Secure airway with tape
14. Administer high-flow oxygen and continue ventilatory assistance as needed
15. Update patient status to hospital and transport immediately

Puncture Method
1. Recognize indications for procedure
2. Select equipment
3. Place a small roll under patient's shoulders to slightly extend neck
4. Locate cricothyroid membrane between the thyroid cartilage and the cricoid cartilage
5. Prepare the skin with antiseptic swab and maintain aseptic technique
6. Stabilize thyroid cartilage between thumb and middle finger of one hand
7. Press index finger of same hand between the thyroid and cricoid cartilage to identify cricothyroid membrane
8. Using index finger as guide
    a. rest middle of ring finger of hand holding needle/cannula on the skin to stabilize and

            prevent needle from penetrating membrane too deeply
- b. make a puncture in the midline with a thrusting motion
- c. insert cannula at a 90° angle
9. After entry into trachea, remove needle, holding cannula in place
10. Check placement of airway by
    - a. ventilating (as necessary) and watching chest rise
    - b. listening for air exchange at the site
    - c. observing patient for color and respiratory improvement
11. Advance cannula into trachea at a 45° angle
12. Tape the cannula securely in place
13. Administer high-flow oxygen or ventilatory assistance as needed
14. Place additional needles/cannulas if needed to assure adequate air exchange
15. Provide update of patient's status to hospital and transport immediately

DEFIBRILLATION

Defibrillation is the application of a direct electrical current to the chest wall of a patient in cardiac arrest. The purpose of this procedure is to convert nonviable arrhythmias to a more life-sustaining pattern. Electrical countershock is not effective in treating asystole even though it is sometimes tried as a last resort.

Do not defibrillate until you have looked at the patient and felt for the pulse, since a loose lead wire or patient movement may mimic ventricular fibrillation. The ability to take a "quick look" through the defibrillator paddles enables you to identify the arrhythmia in less time than it takes to charge the paddles, thereby making blind defibrillation inappropriate.

Select an initial watt/second setting of 200–300 (delivered energy). If unsuccessful immediately defibrillate again with the same watt/second setting. If still unsuccessful, continue CPR and reassess ventilations, give epinephrine 1:10,000 and sodium bicarbonate, and defibrillate again at a setting not to exceed 360 watt/seconds. In children, use a setting of 2 watt/seconds/per kg, not to exceed adult range.

Because the defibrillator delivers a large electrical current, the safety of all personnel involved is as important as the safety of the patient. Defibrillation should be avoided if the patient is very wet or is lying in a puddle of water, as this will disperse the current and endanger both the patient and the paramedic. Burns and arcing of current can be prevented or reduced by using appropriate amounts of saline or gel and firm pressure on the patient's chest. Check to see that everyone is clear of the patient before discharging the current. Personnel providing ventilation and chest compression should continue until the actual time of discharge, when they should pull away momentarily. The person holding the IV line must stand clear of the patient, but will not need to break contact with the IV as the current is not conducted through the line. Because defibrillation induces a seizure of skeletal muscles, the extremity with the IV should be immobilized carefully to prevent dislodgement of the IV line. If you don't see a generalized seizure at the time of defibrillation, you should suspect that the current was inadequate.

When defibrillating children, use special pediatric paddles. If pediatric paddles are not available, the anterior-posterior paddle position is most appropriate. This alternate paddle position is also useful when defibrillating obese or barrel-chested patients, or when normal paddle placement is hampered as by an internal pacemaker.

Immediately following defibrillation reassess the patient and resume CPR if necessary. Response to defibrillation is best evaluated by palpating central pulses and looking for a conversion of the EKG rhythm. Defibrillation most commonly converts ventricular fibrillation into bradycardias, including idioventricular rhythm and supraventricular bradycardias. These arrhythmias can often be improved by using drugs.

Patients in arrest from ventricular fibrillation are assumed to be in concurrent respiratory acidosis. Correction of the acidotic state will improve the potential for conversion of the ventricular arrhythmia. For this reason, sodium bicarbonate can be given prior to defibrillation in an unwitnessed arrest. Epinephrine may also be administered as a means of improving chances of conversion. Lidocaine is indicated during or after the arrest situation to reduce ventricular irritability.

As with all emergency equipment, the defibrillator must always be kept in operational condition. This requires you to check equipment daily to be sure that the battery level is adequate, that all parts are available and that the equipment performs as it should.

PROCEDURAL GUIDELINES	1. Recognize clinical indications for defibrillation
	2. Properly prepare paddles using
	a. gel
	b. saline-soaked pads
	c. commercial pads

3. Turn defibrillator on and select proper w/s setting
4. Press Charge button and wait for unit to reach full charge
5. Demonstrate paddle placement
   a. right: right sternal border, 2nd intercostal space
   b. left: at the apex of the heart
6. Apply paddles with approximately 15 lbs pressure
7. Emphasize safety precautions:
   a. wipe excess gel or saline from the patient
   b. order "stand clear"
   c. keep hands off Discharge button until actual defibrillation
   d. discontinue physical contact with the patient during discharge
8. Simulate defibrillation on a special manikin, or replace paddles in unit and discharge current
9. Check pulses and EKG; order "resume CPR" as needed
10. Report results of defibrillation
11. Discuss variations in technique for:
    a. anterior/posterior paddle placement
    b. pediatric paddles

EKG MONITORING AND TELEMETRY

Electrocardiographic monitoring is the graphic display of the electrical activity of the heart. It is of vital importance in providing effective prehospital management of problems that influence cardiac activity. EKG monitoring should be a priority for those patients with chest pain, difficult breathing, irregular pulse, unconsciousness or profound shock. Monitoring is also done whenever any medication is given that may influence heart rate and rhythm. Monitor the EKG in all questionable situations as a precautionary measure to augment patient assessment.

Remember that good electrode contact is essential. You may need to apply extra gel, dry the diaphoretic patient, shave excess hair or abrade the skin to obtain a good EKG complex. Know how to troubleshoot equipment to alleviate artifact and 60-cycle interference. When faced with a straight-line or what appears to be ventricular fibrillation, check both the patient and the connections to rule out a mechanical problem such as a loose electrode wire. When connecting the cables, assure that electrode wires are attached to the corresponding electrodes or the EKG readout will be inaccurate. Both Leads II and MC1$_1$ are good monitoring leads because they follow the conduction pathways of the heart and therefore show well defined P waves. This allows for easier detection of arrhythmias.

Place the monitor where it is most visible. Watch it closely to detect any abnormalities and anticipate the types of arrhythmias that may occur. Most patients who require EKG monitoring will also require oxygen, IV TKO, and possibly antiarrhythmic medications. Telemetry during cardiac arrest may be done periodically or sometimes continuously to keep the hospital informed of the situation. When sending the EKG via telemetry remember to a) begin with a calibration signal, b) switch your radio mode to EKG and c) allow sufficient time for the hospital to evaluate the rhythm. Avoid interjecting unnecessary voice communications during the EKG transmission as this will distort the cardiac pattern.

PROCEDURAL GUIDELINES

Monitoring

1. Insert lead wires into corresponding patient cable connections
2. Attach chest electrodes
   a. prepare skin
   b. connect electrode wires to electrodes
   c. apply electrodes in correct position on chest wall
3. Attach patient cable to oscilloscope
4. Turn on oscilloscope
5. Select appropriate lead for optimal rhythm interpretation
6. Adjust speed and/or gain if needed
7. Interpret arrhythmias displayed on screen
8. Report arrhythmia interpretation to hospital and request confirmation
9. If monitor has graphic readout, produce a legible rhythm strip
10. Recognize and correct
    - 60-cycle interference
    - loose electrode or wire
    - artifact
    - muscle tremors, patient movement

PROCEDURAL GUIDELINES

Telemetry

1. Attach oscilloscope to radio via connecting

    cable
2. Switch dial on radio from *Voice* to *EKG*
3. Send brief calibration signal to hospital
4. Allow sufficient time for EKG transmission to hospital
5. Identify a rhythm and request verification
6. Identify and correct equipment problems as they arise

ENDOTRACHEAL INTUBATION

Endotracheal (ET) intubation is the insertion of a tube directly into the trachea to open the airway and provide a pathway for ventilatory assistance. An ET tube is indicated in the field when a patient is not breathing effectively, or is not breathing at all. Intubation is contraindicated in upper airway obstruction due to foreign bodies. It should be used with caution in laryngeal edema or in patients with mandibular or cervical fractures, since attempts at intubation may aggravate these conditions.

The major field complication is due to improper placement into the esophagus which in effect forms a total airway obstruction and will result in death if not recognized and corrected. Other immediate complications include aspiration, trauma and/or perforation of the esophagus or pharynx, insertion into the right mainstem bronchus resulting in a left atelectasis, bronchospasm, laryngospasm, hypoxemia, cardiac arrhythmias, and irritation of the carina with subsequent coughing.

Before inserting the airway, position the patient for maximum visual advantage and have suction available. Ventilate with 100% oxygen prior to and following intubation. Have all equipment ready and functioning. Avoid pronounced hyperextension of the neck and never insert the ET tube without direct visualization of the vocal cords. Keep the laryngoscope off the teeth to prevent chipping, which could result in aspiration of tooth fragments by the patient. Once the tube is inserted, inflate the cuff and make sure it is properly positioned by ausculating both lungs for adequate breath sounds. Secure the tube in place with adhesive tape.

PROCEDURAL GUIDELINES

1. Establish need for intubation, i.e., respiratory arrest or inadequate ventilatory exchange
2. Assures that EKG is being monitored
3. Select proper equipment and assure proper functioning
4. Select the appropriate ET tube and lubricate with water-soluble lubricant

5. Have suction and oxygen prepared and available
6. Position patient's head so that trachea and oropharynx are aligned:
   a. place patient in supine position
   b. approach patient's head from above
   c. place pillow or blanket under neck or shoulders
   d. extend head by moving the chin up and back ("sniffing" position)
7. Ventilate with 100% oxygen
8. Grip handle of laryngoscope with left hand so that knuckles are parallel with the blade
9. Insert blade of laryngoscope along the right side of the tongue to its base, and displace the tongue to the left
   a. advance the curved blade to the base of the tongue at the epiglottis, or
   b. advance the straight blade until the tip is under the epiglottis
10. Lift laryngoscope slightly upward and forward with the left hand to extend jaw further:
    a. lift with the shoulder, keeping wrist straight and firm
    b. avoid pressing laryngoscope against patient's teeth
11. Visualize vocal cords
12. Using the right hand, insert the endotracheal tube with its curve facing forward until cuff passes vocal cords
13. Remove the laryngoscope carefully
14. Assure proper placement:
    a. ventilate while auscultating for bilateral lung sounds
    b. watch for chest to rise
15. While ventilating patient, inflate cuff until expired air no longer leaks around cuff, then add 0.5–1 ml more air to assure seal
16. Ventilate with 100% oxygen
17. Insert oropharyngeal airway to act as bite block
18. Securely tape tube in place
19. Continue ventilatory efforts, suctioning as necessary

ESOPHAGEAL OBTURATOR AIRWAY INSERTION

The esophageal obturator airway (EOA) is a cuffed tube which seals off the esophagus and channels ventilated air into the trachea. The concurrent use of a nasogastric (NG) tube either passed through or around the EOA, allows decompression of the stomach and prevents regurgitation. Because the EOA seals off the stomach from the airway, its use during CPR has greatly reduced the incidence of aspiration. Complications associated with use of the EOA include inadvertent intubation of the trachea, and esophageal rupture.

The EOA is indicated in an unconscious, apneic adult. It can be placed blindly without the need to see the oral anatomy and can be inserted with the patient's head in a neutral or slightly flexed position. It is contraindicated in any patient who is conscious because the gag reflex may still be present, and emesis with aspiration may result at the time of insertion. The EOA should not be inserted in a patient with suspected narcotic overdose to whom Narcan will be administered, because the patient is expected to regain consciousness rapidly. It should be used with caution in severe facial trauma or known esophageal disease. Unfortunately, the EOA cannot be used on children because it is not yet available in pediatric sizes.

Before inflating the balloon, assure correct placement by giving one quick breath through the tube and watching for the chest to rise. Auscultate the chest to evaluate adequacy of ventilation. Remove the tube at once if you suspect placement in the trachea. Make sure you have an airtight seal around the mask, and pull the jaw forward for normal airway management. The EOA should not be removed in the field unless the patient actively resists it. Do not remove it without suctioning and positioning the patient to avoid aspiration.

A common problem associated with this procedure is improper removal by personnel who are unfamiliar with its use. To avoid this, make sure all Emergency Department and support personnel are aware of the function and position of the EOA. Endotracheal intubation may be performed with the EOA in place.

PROCEDURAL GUIDELINES

1. Identify indication for EOA insertion
2. Select equipment and assure proper functioning
3. Lubricate tube and attach mask
4. Properly position head in neutral or flexed position
5. Insert tube until mask rests on face (displace tongue laterally and follow curvature of

oropharynx)
6. Check for placement:
   a. make airtight seal with mask
   b. immediately ventilate once through tube, watching for chest to rise, and/or auscultating for air exchange
   c. if intubation is unsuccessful, pull tube out, ventilate and attempt again
   d. once placement is confirmed, inflate cuff with 35 ml air
   e. assess and report patient's status
7. Ventilate patient with supplemental oxygen
   a. maintain airtight seal between mask and face
   b. auscultate chest bilaterally
   c. watch for chest movement
8. Suction oropharynx as needed
9. Pass NG tube as ordered around or through the tube
10. Give indications for removal and demonstrate procedure
    a. turn patient to side
    b. deflate cuff
    c. gently remove tube
    d. use suction as needed
    e. continue supplemental oxygen

INTRACARDIAC INJECTIONS

An intracardiac (IC) injection deposits medication directly into the ventricular chamber of the heart. It is usually performed during cardiac arrest when a standard IV route is unobtainable, or when a direct pharmacological effect on the myocardium is desired. The medications most commonly given as IC injections in the field are Epinephrine and calcium chloride. Because of the potential complications associated with IC injections, there is continuing controversy over its use. However it is still widely used when other resuscitative methods are not possible.

Some degree of myocardial damage probably occurs with every IC injection. Most damage occurs when the heart is still fibrillating or if the needle is jarred during the procedure. The needle tip may tear a coronary artery, the myocardium, or the pericardium. When there is bleeding within the pericardial sac, a pericardial tamponade may develop. Other complications which may be caused by IC injections are hemothorax and pneumothorax.

When performing an IC injection, do not interrupt CPR any longer than necessary. In order to keep the interruption minimal, locate the landmarks for the injection and prepare the medication while CPR is still in progress. Aspirate continuously while advancing the needle through the myocardium. When a free flow of blood appears, inject the medication quickly. Immediately after withdrawing the needle, resume CPR to circulate the drug. Assess the effectiveness of the drug by palpating the pulses and observing the EKG monitor.

Although indications for an IC injection in a child are the same as for an adult, the different anatomical position of the heart in infants and children requires variances in technique. These variances are included in the procedural guidelines.

PROCEDURAL GUIDELINES

1. Identify indications for IC injections
2. Prepare the medication, using aseptic technique
   a. use 3½ inch, 18 gauge needle
   b. withdraw the medication from an ampule or
   c. select a preloaded syringe
3. Recheck drugs, dosage and route
4. Locate injection site and prepare skin
5. Maintaining aseptic technique, insert needle through the skin with a quick thrust
   a. 4th intercostal space, 2 cm left of sternum at a 90° angle
   b. 5th intercostal space, 2 cm left of sternum; aim toward head at a 70°–80° angle
   c. subxiphoid, immediately below and left of xiphoid process; aim toward left shoulder at a 45° angle
6. Advance needle slowly while aspirating
7. When blood flows freely into syringe, quickly inject drug into ventricular cavity
8. Quickly withdraw needle, pressing alcohol swab or gauze over site
9. Direct others to resume CPR
10. Assess effectiveness of medication by evaluating pulse and EKG
11. Report to hospital that drug is "on board" and give patient response

12. Record administration of drug and patient response
13. Demonstrate variations for infants and small children
- infants (newborn to 3 years)
  a. use subxiphoid site only
  b. use 1½-inch 21-gauge needle
  c. insert needle at 20° angle, aiming toward left midclavicular line
- young children (3–12 years)
  a. use 3-inch, 20-gauge needle
  b. subxiphoid or third or fourth intercostal spaces are the only acceptable sites
  c. insert needle
    - subxiphoid, 20° angle, aim for third intercostal space, midclavicular line
    - third intercostal space, 90° angle, straight in
    - fourth intercostal space, aim for head at a 70–80° angle

INTRAMUSCULAR AND SUBCUTANEOUS INJECTIONS

Medications may be injected directly into the patient's tissues either intramuscularly (IM) or subcutaneously (SC). These routes are used when an IV cannot be established, or when a slower absorption rate is preferred over the IV route. Both methods are contraindicated in profound shock states because peripheral circulation is impaired and the drug will remain unabsorbed in the tissues. Complications include nerve damage and local infection, both of which are associated with improper technique.

IM injections are usually given in the deltoid muscle, but may be given into any major muscle mass. Vastus lateralis is the preferred sight in infants. Choose a 21-gauge needle, 1-1½ inches long, and insert the needle at a 90° angle to deposit the drug into the muscle layer. Medications commonly given by the IM route include Benadryl, Valium, atropine sulfate and morphine sulfate.

Subcutaneous injections are given at a 45° angle into the fatty tissues of the upper arm, abdomen or thigh. They require a smaller needle, usually 23-gauge, ⅝ inch. The SC route is used to administer Epinephrine 1:1000 when treating asthma or anaphylaxis, or morphine sulfate.

Before giving any drug, make sure the order includes the route as well as the dosage. Explain the procedure to the patient and ask about allergies. Using aseptic technique, insert the needle quickly, aspirate, inject the drug, and withdraw the needle smoothly. Following the injection, evaluate the patient carefully for both desired and untoward effects.

PROCEDURAL GUIDELINES

Intramuscular (IM) and Subcutaneous (SC) Injections

1. Prepare patient by explaining procedure, checking for allergies, and positioning patient as needed
2. Gather equipment
3. Prepare needle and syringe, maintaining aseptic technique throughout the procedure
4. Withdraw medication from
   a. ampule
   b. vial
      - swab top of vial
      - inject proportional volume of air into bottle and aspirate correct dosage
5. Check for and displace air bubbles prior to injection
6. Select appropriate site
7. Prep skin with antiseptic swab
8. Recheck medication and dosage
9. Properly support skin
10. Insert needle with bevel up
    - IM injections, needle should be at a 90° angle
    - SC injections, needle should be at a 45° angle
11. Release skin before injecting solution
12. Aspirate to ensure needle is not in a blood vessel
13. Inject solution slowly and smoothly
14. Support skin with antiseptic swab while quickly withdrawing needle
15. Massage skin to help with absorption of drug
16. Report that drug is "on board"
17. Monitor and report patient's response to drug
18. Record time and site of injection on prehospital report form

IV INSERTION INTO THE EXTERNAL JUGULAR VEIN

An IV catheter may be inserted into the external jugular vein in order to infuse various medications and IV solutions into the circulatory system. This route is selected only after other peripheral IV attempts have been unsuccessful and an IV line is essential to patient management.

The external jugular vein is a large peripheral vessel which runs superficially along the side of the neck between the ear and the midclavicular line. It can be distended by a) compressing the vein immediately above the clavicle, b) lowering the head, and/or c) elevating the lower extremities if the patient is in severe circulatory collapse.

Complications which may occur from external jugular cannulation include air embolism, pneumothorax, hematoma and infiltration. Air embolus can be avoided by placing the patient in a Trendelenberg position, clearing the IV tubing of air, and firmly tamponading the vein while connecting the tubing to the cannula. To help prevent pneumothorax, puncture the vein as closely as possible to the angle of the jaw. Watch closely for signs of hematoma formation or infiltration. If either occurs, discontinue the IV and apply firm pressure.

Following the procedure, auscultate the lungs frequently to detect the occurrence of pneumothorax or fluid overload. Tape the cannula securely to avoid possible dislodgement caused by patient movement.

PROCEDURAL GUIDELINES

1. Gather equipment
2. Place patient in supine position, with head lowered slightly and turned at a 45°–60° angle from the midline
3. Locate external jugular vein
4. Cleanse skin thoroughly with antiseptic swabs
5. Stabilize the skin above proposed puncture site by using gentle countertraction
6. Distend vein by
   a. compressing just above clavicle
   b. lowering patient's head
   c. elevating lower extremities
7. Using aseptic technique, make venipuncture midway between the angle of the jaw and the midclavicular line.
8. Make first thrust lateral to vein to penetrate the skin
9. Once through the skin, adjust angle and can-

nulate vein itself, while aspirating for blood return

10. When vein has been penetrated, remove needle and advance cannula
11. As cannula is inserted, compress vein at end of catheter.
12. Draw blood if ordered, maintaining compression on vein while removing the syringe
13. Connect IV tubing *securely* to cannula end and release compression
14. Set IV flow rate as ordered and adjust as needed
15. Tape needle (or catheter) and tubing securely in place
16. Check IV site frequently
17. Auscultate lung sounds to rule out pneumothorax and fluid overload
18. Report completed cannulation to hospital
19. Record site, time, and needle size on prehospital report form
20. Explain variations for infants and children
    a. have assistant support child's head and neck over edge of table while securing shoulders firmly on the table
    b. mummy-wrap wriggling infants if necessary

IV INSERTION INTO PERIPHERAL VEIN

The insertion of an indwelling catheter into a vein is done to establish direct access into the circulatory system. This line can then be used to administer specific medications or replace intravenous fluids. The vein is often cannulated just in case medications are needed.

The site for an IV varies according to the patient's veins and clinical condition. Ideally, the most distal veins of the upper extremities should be used first so that other veins are available if repeated cannulations are necessary. In life-threatening emergencies, the larger veins of the antecubital fossa can be used because of their easy access.

The size and type of IV needle/cannula you select will vary with the size of the patient's veins, the clinical indication for the IV, and to a small degree, your individual preference. Use large-bore cannulas in hypovolemic conditions when fluid replacement is needed. The smaller scalp vein needles can be used for children, elderly patients with fragile veins and TKO IV's. Cannulas are generally preferred over scalp-vein needles because they are less likely to infiltrate.

To facilitate venous distension, apply a constricting band, lower the extremity, and/or stroke the vein upward. With difficult veins, the application of heat or an ace wrap may further distend the vein.

To stabilize the vein during the puncture, insert the needle at a bifurcation and/or apply countertraction and anchor the vein with your fingers. Secure the cannula or needle but avoid taping around the entire extremity as this may create a tourniquet effect if infiltration occurs. Use an arm board whenever the IV has been started near a joint.

If the IV begins to flow poorly or there is redness, pain, or swelling around the IV site, suspect infiltration and restart the IV as needed. Throughout the procedure, use aseptic technique to reduce the occurrence of local and systemic infections. To prevent air embolism, clear the tubing of air initially and assure that all connections are tightly secured.

Closely watch the IV drip rate, especially after giving an IV medication or changing the patient's position. Auscultate lung sounds frequently and reduce the IV flow if pulmonary congestion develops.

PROCEDURAL GUIDELINES

1. Gather and prepare equipment
2. Apply a constricting band and assess peripheral pulse
3. Identify an appropriate vein
4. If necessary, produce additional venous distension by one or more of the following:
   a. tapping the vein
   b. stroking the vein upward
   c. lowering the extremity
5. Prep site with antiseptic swab; maintain aseptic technique throughout procedure
6. Stabilize vein
   a. use fingers to apply countertraction
   b. insert needle at bifurcation when possible
7. Puncture vein with
   • cannula over needle
   a. pierce skin at a 20° angle on top of or along side the vein
   b. adjust angle of insertion to enter vein
   c. watch or aspirate for flashback of blood
   d. advance cannula and remove needle
   • scalp vein needle
   a. pierce skin at a 20° angle on top of or along

   side the vein
   b. adjust angle of insertion to enter vein
   c. watch or aspirate for flashback of blood
   d. advance needle into vein
8. Tamponade above the puncture site to reduce bleeding
9. Connect IV tubing firmly to cannula/scalp vein
10. Release constricting band
11. Start IV flow and check for infiltration
12. Secure IV by
    a. applying tape
    b. applying armboard as needed
13. Recheck IV flow rate, and adjust as needed
14. Evaluate patient's lung sounds and respiratory rate
15. Report IV initiation
16. Reassess IV for patency and drip rate
17. Record site, time, and needle/cannula size on prehospital report form

IV INSERTION INTO THE SUBCLAVIAN VEIN

A catheter may be inserted into the subclavian vein to provide access for IV fluids and/or medications. The subclavian site for IV initiation has the following advantages over peripheral sites: 1) it is a large central vein; 2) it provides for quick absorption of medications; 3) it handles a large volume of fluid easily, and 4) it allows for easy insertion of a transvenous pacemaker wire if needed. This site is used when a peripheral line is not possible or in cardiac arrest situations.

This procedure can produce severe complications such as hemothorax, pneumothorax, and lacerated veins or arteries. To help prevent pneumothorax, instruct the alert patient to take shallow breaths during the procedure. In addition, avoid inserting the needle too deeply, or entering the vein at the wrong angle, or changing the angle of the needle carelessly.

Another major complication is air embolism. There are four ways to help prevent this complication: 1) place the patient in Trendelenberg position; 2) tamponade the catheter following removal of the needle; 3) keep all IV line connections secure, and 4) assure that all air is removed from the IV line.

Prepare the skin well to reduce the incidence of infection. Once the cannula is in place, tape it securely and prevent excessive patient movement. If there is too much movement of the IV cannula, it can be displaced, causing severe bleeding into the thorax. Lung sounds should be auscultated following the procedure to rule out a pneumothorax. If this is suspected, transport the patient promptly.

Following correct placement, adjust the IV rate and monitor the patient closely for possible fluid overload since the subclavian vein is very large and can accommodate a large volume of fluid very rapidly.

PROCEDURAL GUIDELINES

1. Gather equipment
2. Prepare patient and explain procedure (if conscious)
3. Position patient
   a. supine
   b. Trendelenberg
   c. turn head to opposite side of puncture
   d. place pillow under shoulders (optional)
4. Prepare area with antiseptic swab (mid-sternum lateral to shoulder joint, including suprasternal notch)
5. Instruct alert patient to take shallow breaths
6. Insert cannula, using aseptic technique 1 cm below the midclavicular point at 10°–15° angle to skin
7. Advance cannula slowly toward upper border of suprasternal notch
8. Assess entrance into vein by observing a free flow of blood into cannula
9. Advance cannula to thread it into vein
10. Tamponade end of cannula, quickly pull out needle and connect IV tubing to cannula
11. Tape cannula securely in place and apply dressing
12. Establish drip rate
13. Auscultate chest, and observe for complications
14. Report completion of procedure and patient status
15. Record site, time and needle size on prehospital report forms

IV MEDICATION ADMINISTRATION

Medications administered intravenously are injected directly into the vascular system. The intravenous (IV) route is preferred when an immediate response is needed in such life threatening situations as cardiac and/or respiratory arrest, or when peripheral circulation is impaired, as with myocardial infarction, shock, and drug overdose. While most IV medications are injected via an indwelling IV line, they may also be given directly into a vein or infused gradually after being diluted in a Volutrol or in a bag of IV solution. The method of administration will vary according to the properties of the specific medication and the desired effect on an individual patient.

Before injecting any IV medication, ensure that infiltration has not occurred. Infiltration will impede absorption, and in some instances may cause tissue necrosis.

Since the IV route provides rapid distribution of the medication, therapeutic actions as well as side effects will occur quickly. Therefore, it is essential to monitor the patient's response closely. Before administering any drug, check the patient's history for drug allergies and make sure the drug is not outdated. Verify drug orders with the hospital, prepare and administer doses accurately, evaluate responses, and record all drug administrations on the patient's record. Question any order which appears inappropriate, and withhold administration of the drug if the question cannot be resolved.

PROCEDURAL GUIDELINES

Direct IV Push

1. Question patient regarding allergies
2. Identify medication to be given by name, dosage and route
3. Prepare prescribed medication by assembling a preloaded syringe, or drawing the appropriate dose from an ampule or vial
4. Apply a constricting band and select a vein
5. Prepare puncture site with antiseptic swab; maintain aseptic technique throughout procedure
6. After rechecking medication and dosage, insert needle at a 10° angle to the skin and advance into vein
7. Aspirate for blood return
8. Remove tourniquet
9. Inject medication at appropriate rate, aspirating at intervals to ensure that needle remains in vein
10. Remove the needle and compress site to prevent formation of hematoma
11. Report to hospital that drug is "on board"

12. Assess and report patient's response
13. Record time of administration on prehospital report form

IV Push via IV Line
1. Question patient regarding allergies
2. Identify medication to be given by name, dosage and route
3. Prepare prescribed medication by assembling a preloaded syringe, or drawing appropriate dose from an ampule or vial
4. Select injection site on IV tubing closest to patient and wipe with antiseptic swab
5. Recheck medication and dosage; ensure IV is not infiltrated, administer through IV injection site, maintaining aseptic technique
    a. for large volumes, pinch off IV flow above injection site; for small volumes, allow IV to continue dripping
    b. inject drug at proper rate
    c. readjust drip rate as needed
6. Report to hospital that drug is "on board"
7. Assess and report patient's response
8. Record time of administration on prehospital report form

IV Volutrol
1. Question patient regarding allergies
2. Identify medication to be given by name, dosage and route
3. Set up an IV bag using a Volutrol administration set
    a. fill Volutrol with desired amount of solution
    b. close valve between IV bag and Volutrol
    c. open air vent
4. Add medication to Volutrol
    a. wipe injection site with with antiseptic swab
    b. recheck medication and dosage and inject drug through injection site on Volutrol
    c. run solution through drip chamber and tubing

    d. label Volutrol with medication, dosage and time

5. Piggyback this IV set into main IV line and secure with tape; close clamp on main IV tubing
6. Regulate drip rate by adjusting flow-regulation clamp below Volutrol
7. Evaluate patient during administration
8. When volume has been infused, report drug is "on board"
9. Shut off flow on Volutrol tubing and re-establish IV flow on main IV line
10. Record drug administration and patient response on prehospital report form

IV Drip

1. Question patient regarding allergies
2. Identify medication to be given by name, dosage and route; prepare as necessary
3. Set up a new IV bag, with tubing attached but not filled
4. Wipe injection site on bag with antiseptic swab
5. Recheck medication and dosage and inject it into IV bag while maintaining aseptic technique
6. Label bag with medication, dosage, date and time
7. Squeeze or tilt bag to mix medication; fill tubing
8. Piggyback this IV into main IV line and secure it in place with tape; close clamp on main IV tubing
9. Adjust flow to specified rate, or titrate to pulse or blood pressure
10. Assess patient's vital signs (including lung sounds) frequently
11. Report to hospital
    a. IV solution in progress
    b. rate of infusion
    c. patient's response to medication
12. Record drug information and patient response on prehospital report form

IV SET-UP

The selection and preparation of IV equipment is essential prior to cannulation of the vein. To save time when initiating an IV, use another member of your team to prepare the set-up while you select the insertion site. Specify which equipment you need assembled.

Select the IV administration set depending upon the desired rate of infusion. The standard maxidrip set administers one ml in 10–20 drops and is used for volume replacement. The microdrip set delivers one ml in 60 drops and is safer to use whenever a controlled infusion rate is required. Add extension tubing to the IV administration set as needed.

A Volutrol or similar volume control chamber is an important measure in controlling fluid intake in very young, old, or critically ill patients who cannot tolerate a large volume of fluids. It is also necessary for diluting certain drugs in the field. The Volutrol may come as a part of the IV administration set (usually with a microdrip) or it may be added to the set-up between the bag and tubing.

Before administering an IV, check each solution container for leaks, obvious contamination, and expiration date. The Viaflex bags have several advantages over bottles, as they can be manually compressed to increase the IV flow rate and are unbreakable. However, caution must be used to prevent puncturing the bag. The manufacturer warns that marking with a felt pen directly on the bag can contaminate the solution, so use an adhesive label instead.

PROCEDURAL GUIDELINES

1. Gather equipment and select appropriate IV administration set
2. Maintain aseptic technique throughout the procedure
3. Remove IV solution bag from outer wrapping
   a. check expiration date
   b. check bag for leakage or cloudy solution
   c. remove tab from port for IV tubing insertion
4. Prepare the IV set by closing drip regulator below drip chamber, and uncapping spiked end of IV tubing
5. Firmly insert spike of IV administration set into port of IV bag to pierce diaphragm
6. Fill IV tubing with fluid.
   a. squeeze drip chamber to fill it no more than half way
   b. open drip regulator to allow fluid to fill rest

of the tubing
   c. uncap distal end of tubing to evacuate air
      from tubing as necessary
   d. recap tubing to maintain sterility
7. Ensure that all air has been evacuated from
   tubing
8. Insert IV extension tubing and/or stopcock at
   distal end of IV administration set and flush
   with IV fluid.

MAGILL FORCEPS

The Magill forceps and laryngoscope are instruments used for removing
an object obstructing the upper airway. This procedure intervenes in a life-
threatening emergency; therefore, you must perform it rapidly and without delay. The laryngoscope provides illumination of the posterior
oropharynx, which allows you to view the obstruction. The Magill forceps
are then used to grasp and remove the foreign matter. Use this procedure
only on an *unconscious* patient and in conjunction with other maneuvers
for airway obstruction, i.e., back blows and manual thrusts.

Complications include laryngospasm, soft tissue damage, and chipped
teeth. Avoid these complications by exercising caution when inserting and
removing these instruments. Particularly avoid resting the laryngoscope
blade on the teeth. Check the laryngoscope daily to ensure that the battery
and bulb are operational.

Manage the patient with high flow oxygen, cardiac monitoring and
suctioning as needed.

PROCEDURAL
GUIDELINES

1. Approach supine patient's head from above.
2. Hyperextend patient's head and neck unless
   contraindicated
3. Insert a bite stick, if feasible
4. Insert laryngoscope
   a. grasp handle with left hand, so that
      knuckles are parallel to blade
   b. place blade of laryngoscope to the right of
      tongue and displace tongue to left
   c. pull slightly up and out in direction of
      handle, extending jaw further
5. Visualize foreign object
6. Hold Magill forceps in right hand, palm
   down, with closed tips curving down

7. Insert closed tips of forceps down to object; be careful not to push the object further down into the airway

8. Open tips and clamp them firmly around object (If object cannot be grasped with tips of forceps, deflect object to one side to open airway)

9. Remove object by carefully pulling forceps out

10. Remove laryngoscope carefully (reverse insertion procedure)

11. When object has been removed (or displaced to one side) reassess lung sounds, and continue with airway management.

NASOGASTRIC INTUBATION

A nasogastric (NG) tube is inserted into the stomach via the nose to relieve distension caused by foods, fluids, blood or air. If left uncorrected, the increased intraabdominal pressure can cause vomiting and subsequent aspiration, bradycardia, or decreased lung expansion. This procedure is used in the treatment of near drowning, cardiac arrest, upper GI hemorrhage, drug overdose and poisonings.

Lubricate the NG tube generously to facilitate passage. Place the patient in high Fowler's position and advance the tube while he/she swallows or sips small amounts of water. If the patient doesn't swallow, gently stroke downward on his/her throat to stimulate the swallowing reflex. Monitor the patient closely while inserting the NG tube since vagal stimulation may induce arrhythmias.

Once the tube has been inserted, verify proper placement by aspirating for stomach contents. If no contents are aspirated, inject a bolus of air and listen over epigastrium. Watch for coughing, hoarse speech, cyanosis or dyspnea, any of which might indicate misplacement of the tube into the trachea. If this occurs, remove the tube and attempt reinsertion.

The gastric contents may be aspirated manually or attached to intermittent suction. If continuous suction is all that is available, use a vented NG tube to avoid trauma to the stomach lining.

Occasionally the NG tube might become obstructed or wedged against the stomach lining, thereby necessitating irrigation or repositioning. Any aspirated contents should be saved for analysis at the hospital.

PROCEDURAL GUIDELINES

1. Select equipment
2. Explain procedure and position patient

3. Measure insertion length from nose to ear to xiphoid and mark with tape
4. Lubricate tube
5. Attach tube to irrigating syringe
6. Slowly and gently insert NG tube through nares as patient swallows
7. Evaluate placement by aspirating for stomach contents; if no contents are aspirated, inject air into the tube and listen over epigastrium with a stethoscope
8. Attach tube to suction, if indicated
9. Tape tube securely in position; avoid pressure on nares; avoid uncomfortable or inconvenient taping
10. Proceed with aspiration or irrigation as directed

PERICARDIOCENTESIS

Pericardiocentesis is the insertion of a needle into the pericardial sac to remove accumulated blood. It is the treatment of choice for cardiac tamponade, a condition wherein blood and/or fluid accumulate in the pericardial space and quickly suppress the heart's pumping action. This condition usually results from blunt chest trauma and must be alleviated immediately to prevent circulatory collapse and death.

Cardiac tamponade should be suspected whenever a patient with chest trauma continues to deteriorate despite aggressive therapy. Signs indicating rapid development of tamponade may include muffled or inaudible heart sounds, tachycardia, hypotension, distended neck veins, paradoxical pulse, or signs of profound shock.

When performing a pericardiocentesis, it is important to determine correct landmarks and closely observe the angle of insertion to facilitate entry into the pericardium. Complications that may occur include lacerated coronary artery, ventricular tear, and pneumothorax. Avoid inserting the needle too deeply, as blood might then be aspirated from the ventricle rather than the pericardium. If the first attempt is unsuccessful, repeat the procedure until some fluid can be removed. Normal cardiac output may be restored if even as little as 30 ml can be withdrawn.

Administer high-flow oxygen concurrently, but avoid positive pressure ventilation if possible because it will elevate the intrathoracic pressure. Monitor and auscultate the chest frequently to assess patient status and determine additional treatment.

PROCEDURAL GUIDELINES

1. Identify indication for procedure
2. Prepare equipment; use a 3½ inch, 18 gauge needle attached to a 3 ml syringe
3. Prepare the patient by applying cardiac monitor, inserting an IV line, and placing patient in a supine position at 60° angle
4. Locate proper injection site, i.e., immediately below left rib cage and slightly to left of xiphoid process
5. Prep skin with antiseptic swab
6. Using aseptic technique, slowly insert the needle 8–10 cm at a 45° angle to the skin; aim toward right sternoclavicular joint; aspirate while inserting
7. Stop inserting needle when blood is aspirated
8. Aspirate available blood, changing syringes if necessary
9. Withdraw needle and apply pressure to puncture site
10. Evaluate patient for improvement in cardiac output and report to hospital
11. Transport immediately in position of comfort, continuing high flow oxygen

ROTATING TOURNIQUETS

Rotating tourniquets are constricting bands placed on the extremities of a patient experiencing acute distress from pulmonary edema. They temporarily trap enough blood in the extremities to significantly diminish venous return to the right side of the heart. This procedure helps reduce cardiac workload and lung congestion, thereby alleviating signs of acute distress such as rales, dyspnea and shortness of breath.

Rotating tourniquets are used concurrently with high-flow oxygen, positive-pressure ventilation, and drugs such as morphine sulfate, Lasix, and Aminophylline. Place the tourniquets as high on the extremities as possible to obtain maximum benefit. Do not place a tourniquet on the extremity to which the IV is connected, as that will occlude the flow. Be sure to assess all peripheral pulses after application. Rotate the tourniquets clockwise every 15 minutes and accurately record their placement. Monitor EKG to detect cardiac arrhythmias, and auscultate lungs frequently to assess respiratory changes. If ordered to discontinue this procedure, remove one tourniquet every fifteen minutes. Never remove all tourniquets at once because this will cause sudden engorgement of the heart and lungs, with subsequent deterioration of the patient's condition.

PROCEDURAL GUIDELINES

1. Identify indications for rotating tourniquets
2. Explain procedure to patient
3. Gather equipment
4. Apply tourniquet snugly to:
   a. 3 of 4 extremities, if no IV established
   b. 2 of 3 extremities, if IV established
   c. place tourniquets high on upper arms and thighs
5. Assure that arterial pulses are palpable distal to tourniquets
6. Note time of application and record placement clearly, using stick figures to show positioning of tourniquets
7. Rotate tourniquets clockwise every 15 minutes
   a. apply tourniquet to "open" extremity
   b. remove appropriate tourniquet
   c. record timing and rotation pattern accurately
   d. reevaluate pulses
   e. continue pattern of rotation until ordered to discontinue
8. If ordered to terminate procedure, remove one tourniquet every 15 minutes
9. Assess and report patient's response to procedure

SUCTIONING

Suctioning is used to remove obstructive substances from the respiratory tract with an external suction source. It can be used to stimulate coughing to remove secretions from the distal airways. Conditions in which suctioning may be indicated include unconsciousness, near drowning, organophosphate poisoning, facial trauma and vomiting. Additionally, any patient who is intubated usually requires suctioning. The two methods of suctioning are oropharyngeal and tracheal.

Oropharyngeal suctioning is usually accomplished with a tonsil-tip catheter. This is not a sterile procedure since the trachea is not entered. Tonsil tip suctioning is a quick and easy method for clearing the oropharynx of large particles such as blood and vomitus. When using the tonsil tip it is important to remember not to push the tip of the catheter too deep into the oropharynx as this may stimulate a gag reflex. If the tonsil tip catheter is not available or if the vomitus or food particles are too large to pass through the tonsil tip, the end of the suction connecting tubing can be used.

Tracheal suctioning can be accomplished by passing a suction catheter either through the nares or through an endotracheal tube into the trachea. This procedure is performed using sterile technique to prevent the introduction of pathogens into the respiratory tract. The patient who requires tracheal suctioning is usually hypoxic before the procedure has begun. This hypoxia is compounded by the use of suction, which draws off available oxygen. To reduce this problem, hyperoxygenate the patient prior to and following the procedure, and keep suctioning intervals as brief as possible.

Tracheal suctioning may stimulate the vagus nerve and cause reflex bradycardia. Temporarily discontinue suctioning if this occurs and perform subsequent attempts with caution. Damage to the mucous membrane is another complication. The possibility of this occurring can be reduced by a) avoiding force when passing the catheter, b) lubricating the nasal catheter well, and c) assuring that the suction source is off during insertion of the catheter. Monitor the patient closely during the procedure, give oxygen liberally, and assess the respiratory status regularly to determine the need for further suctioning.

PROCEDURAL GUIDELINES

Oropharyngeal Suctioning

1. Select equipment
2. Inform patient
3. Position patient on side to facilitate drainage
4. Connect tonsil tip catheter to suction tubing
5. While applying intermittent suction, run the catheter tip along the gum line and across tongue
6. Assess and report patient's response to procedure

Tracheal Suctioning

1. Select equipment
2. Inform patient
3. Give patient presuctioning oxygen
4. Position patient in high Fowler's position if conscious; in a supine position if unconscious

5. Connect catheter to suction tubing
6. Lubricate catheter tip
7. With suction off, insert catheter through nares or endotracheal tube until patient coughs
8. Apply suction intermittently, rotating as you withdraw it
9. Oxygenate patient and allow short rest period
10. Reinsert catheter and repeat process, if needed
11. Suction individual bronchi if necessary by turning patient's head to alternate sides before inserting catheter
12. Observe patient for hypoxia or bradyarrhythmias and delay procedure as indicated
13. Assess and report patient's response to procedure

THORACOSTOMY (NEEDLE)

A needle thoracostomy is a procedure in which an opening is made in the thorax to relieve a tension pneumothorax. Tension pneumothorax is a condition which occurs when air enters the pleural space through a tear in the lung, but is prevented from exiting by a tissue flap that creates a one-way valve effect. The pleural space is inflated with each expiration, subsequently preventing complete lung expansion. If the condition is allowed to persist it can eventually cause collapse of the lung, displacement of the trachea and mediastinum, and finally bilateral pneumothorax with resultant respiratory collapse.

Signs indicating tension pneumothorax include increasing dyspnea with cyanosis and shock, decreased or absent breath sounds, distended neck veins, and tracheal deviation.

Diagnosis of tension pneumothorax is often difficult to make, and to perform a needle thoracostomy in the absence of tension pneumothorax can induce a pneumothorax and/or hemothorax. Although tension pneumothorax can be fatal if left untreated, it rarely progresses to a life-threatening stage in less time than it takes to transport the patient. Therefore, it may be more appropriate to transport the patient than to initiate invasive field treatment unless the transport time would be unusually long. If it is determined that the patient is, in fact, suffering from tension pneumothorax and requires immediate relief, a needle thoracostomy may be ordered.

A needle thoracostomy is performed by inserting a large-bore cannula needle into the pleural cavity to reduce the intrathoracic pressure. A rapid rush of air from the cannula indicates entry into the pleural space, thus relieving the tension. Once this occurs, a one-way flutter valve (such as a Heimlich valve) is used to allow air to escape while preventing further air from entering the pleural cavity. A combination needle/one-way valve (such as the McSwain Dart) might be available to expedite the procedure.

Following the procedure, transport the patient immediately, monitoring vital signs and patient status frequently enroute. Continue ventilatory support with high-flow oxygen and position patient to facilitate air exchange.

PROCEDURAL GUIDELINES

1. Identify signs and symptoms indicating a tension pneumothorax
2. Gather equipment
3. Properly locate landmarks on the side of the tension pneumothorax
   a. 2nd intercostal space at midclavicular line, or
   b. 4th or 5th intercostal space at mid-axillary line
4. Prep skin with an antiseptic swab
5. Using aseptic technique, insert cannula at a 90° angle at superior border of rib, approximately 1½ inches into pleural space
7. Remove needle from cannula; ensure that flutter valve is firmly attached to cannula
   a. connect valve and cannula if separate
   b. check connection if pre-attached
8. Secure cannula and flutter valve to chest wall with tape
9. Report patient's response to procedure
10. Transport immediately in position of comfort and continue high-flow oxygen
11. Frequently update vital signs, lung sounds, and patient status

TRIAGE

The role of the paramedic in a multiple casualty incident is primarily sophisticated assessment, direction of patient management, and basic life support. Advanced life support is only appropriate if there are small numbers of patients.

In the multi-casualty situation you must consider the number of patients, available personnel, extent and severity of injuries, and the ages and medical conditions of the patients in order to determine the complexity of the situation and set priorities to manage it.

After assessing the scene and the capabilities of your team, you must exercise leadership and respond with appropriate degree of urgency, judgment, and skill to deal with the problems at hand. Call for backup as soon as the need is identified and contact the hospital to request authority to operate under disaster protocols.

In a multiple-patient incident, it is essential that a single individual be identified as triage officer to direct patient management without confusion and duplication. The first-in paramedic is usually in the best position to accept this responsibility. In this role the paramedic assigned to the radio (radio person) will direct all other patient care personnel, communicate with the hospital, and coordinate all patient management. Make sure the directions you give to other rescue personnel are clear and concise; leave no room for misunderstandings.

The paramedic triage officer is also responsible for requesting additional medical support such as regional triage teams if necessary. Once a triage team arrives, the physician will assume the role of triage officer and will then direct all prehospital care.

A nonmedical person, usually the highest ranking fire department official, controls the nonmedical aspects of the scene. This person will be responsible for scene safety, coordination of ambulances and other emergency vehicles, fire suppression, crowd control, and rescue activities.

On arrival at a multi-casualty incident, set up a communications base in a safe place near access to ambulances. If the patients are scattered, have them gathered to a central location. The radio person, accompanied by other rescue personnel, must immediately perform a 30-second survey of each patient, identify the most life-threatening injuries, and direct other personnel to institute appropriate measures with that patient. In order to minimize confusion, only the radio person should communicate with the hospital. Compile a separate record for each patient and use it to organize radio reports. Report on the most serious patients first, using ID numbers for clarity. In triage situations, field treatment is generally confined to ABCs and rarely gets more sophisticated than an IV and/or antishock trousers. Be certain that all treatment records are securely affixed to the patient.

Each patient is assigned a priority for care and/or transportation. Prioritization categories vary across the country but all of them incorporate the principle of doing the most good for the most people. The following is one example of triage categories:

1. *Urgent Intervention*

Patients with an urgent medical problem which requires minimal intervention to stabilize. Examples include airway obstruction, isolated bleeding.

2. *Immediate Transport*
   Patients with major injuries requiring sophisticated treatment not available in the field, thereby necessitating immediate transport. Examples include major head, chest or abdominal trauma or multi-system injuries.

3. *Walking Wounded*
   Patients with minor injuries whose need for care/transport is not immediate and may even be able to assist in their own care or the care of others. Examples include sprains, minor fractures, small cuts, abrasions.

4. *Delayed Treatment*
   Patients with a low probability for resuscitation and/or whose needs are so extensive that care would monopolize your resources. These patients are attended to only after other patients are treated, or if additional personnel become available. For example, cardiac arrest associated with trauma, dead.

Have the hospital inventory available resources and direct patients to hospitals capable of handling their specific injuries. In preparing to transport, fill each ambulance according to the capabilities of the facility it is going to. For example, if ambulance A is going to a hospital which has a trauma center and a burn unit, those patients with major trauma and/or burns should be placed in ambulance A, rather than ambulance B, which is going to a small community hospital with limited resources and no surgical staff available. Ambulance B should be filled with patients in the ambulatory category, who will be most likely to receive adequate care at the smaller hospital.

Triage Officer

PROCEDURAL GUIDELINES

1. Recognize existence of a multiple-patient incident and determine safety of the scene
2. Assess scene to determine number of patients, need for additional personnel/resources and obtain authority to operate under disaster protocols
3. Call for backup as soon as the need is identified; call for regional triage team if necessary
4. Set up communications base in a safe place near the ambulances
5. Have patients gathered to central location
6. Perform a 30-second survey of each patient

    a. direct patient care personnel to correct urgent medical problems
    b. assign ID number
    c. assign priority for care and transportation
7. Compile a separate record for each patient; use when communicating information
8. Delegate, coordinate, and oversee care given by others
    a. restrict care to ABC's, IV, antishock measures
    b. adjust care according to available resources and demands of total patient population
    c. ensure that treatment records are securely affixed to patient
9. Assign patients to ambulances according to capabilities of hospital to which they are going

VAGOTONIC MANEUVERS

Stimulation of the vagus nerve causes slowing of the sinus node and decreases conduction through the AV junction. Therefore, in supraventricular tachycardias, vagal stimulation is frequently an effective method of slowing or even converting these arrhythmias to a more adequate pattern. Any method of vagal stimulation should be performed in the prehospital setting only if the patient is experiencing signs and symptoms of decreased cardiac output caused by the supraventricular tachycardia.

There are two forms of vagal stimulation commonly used in the field, Valsalva's maneuver and carotid sinus massage. Both of these methods can be potentially lethal. Prior to attempting any vagotonic maneuver, administer oxygen, start an IV TKO and monitor the EKG. Have full resuscitative equipment ready and inform the patient of the procedure. Monitor vital signs before, during, and after the procedure.

Valsalva's maneuver is the most convenient of these mechanisms. It is performed by having the patient take a deep breath and bear down against the closed glottis, much like straining for a bowel movement. Although this appears to be a simple procedure, it can cause severe bradyarrhythmias including asystole, so monitor the EKG very closely. If Valsalva's maneuver doesn't convert the arrhythmia, carotid sinus massage may be necessary.

Carotid sinus massage (CSM) is a noninvasive method of stimulating the vagus nerve. Because vagus nerve endings are located in the carotid sinus, external pressure to the neck at the site of the carotid sinus can cause the heart rate to decrease. Extreme caution must be used in performing this procedure as it can result in severe bradycardias, asystole, or cerebral vascular disorders. Prior to performing carotid sinus massage, you must check for equality of carotid pulses and avoid massaging a side with a diminished pulse. Initially attempt to convert the rhythm by firm pressure alone. If this is ineffective, proceed to cautiously massage the carotid sinus. Massage only one side at a time, and discontinue massage at the first signs of a slowing rhythm. Do not massage for more than 5–10 seconds, and stop immediately if the patient shows signs of dizziness or other response.

When performing any vagotonic maneuver, monitor the EKG throughout the procedure. Rhythms that may follow vagal stimulation include bradycardias, heart blocks, ventricular tachycardia, ventricular fibrillation, and asystole. Cerebral complications may include syncope, convulsions, or hemiplegia. Increased parasympathetic tone may produce hypotension, nausea, vomiting, or bronchospasm.

If vagal stimulation is unsuccessful in slowing or converting the rhythm, digoxin, Inderal or even cardioversion may be necessary.

Several other mechanisms, including the "diving seal" reflex and the orbital pressure maneuver, are also known to produce slowing of the heart rate. However, they have not been demonstrated to have an appropriate application in the prehospital setting, and have therefore been omitted from this discussion. It is also noted that vomiting has a vagotonic effect, and is often followed by a reflex bradycardia. However, induced vomiting may cause aspiration; therefore its use is not recommended.

PROCEDURAL GUIDELINES

1. Give indications for vagal stimulation
2. Check to see that patient has oxygen and an IV, and is on a cardiac monitor
3. Explain the procedure to the patient
4. Prepare resuscitative equipment
5. Instruct patient to perform Valsalva's maneuver
   a. have patient take a deep breath and bear down
   b. maintain this maneuver for 5–10 seconds or until first sign of slowing of heart, or until first sign of dizziness or decreasing level of consciousness
6. If no response to Valsalva's maneuver, proceed with CSM
7. Place patient in a supine position with head hyperextended; check for equality of carotid

pulses, then rotate head to expose appropriate carotid sinus

8. Properly locate carotid sinus at intersection of
   a. straight line down from ear to clavicle
   b. straight line back from larynx
9. Using flat side of 2–3 fingers, press firmly over carotid sinus
10. If no response, massage carotid sinus by pressing firmly toward cervical vertebrae and massaging up and back in a circular motion
11. Discontinue the procedure
    a. after 5–10 seconds, or
    b. at first sign of a slowing heart rate, or
    c. if patient experiences dizziness or altered level of consciousness
12. Repeat procedure once on opposite side if necessary and not contraindicated
13. Evaluate and report patient's response

VENIPUNCTURE

Venipuncture refers generally to the insertion of a needle into a vein. As used here, venipuncture means drawing a blood sample. In the prehospital setting, a blood sample is necessary to document baseline blood sugar levels prior to administration of glucose to diabetics or unconscious patients.

The primary complication from venipuncture is hematoma formation due to failure to compress the site after the needle has been removed. Avoid unnecessary venipuncture in hemophiliacs or patients on anticoagulants, since excessive bleeding may follow. If an IV line is also being established, a blood sample can be drawn at that time to avoid the need for an additional venipuncture.

Be sure to support the extremity during the procedure. Stabilize the vein to prevent it from rolling. Fill the tubes completely and label each with the proper patient information.

PROCEDURAL GUIDELINES

Venipuncture Using Needle and Syringe
1. Gather equipment
2. Identify an appropriate site (usually antecubital fossa)

3. Apply a constricting band proximal to site and distend vein
4. Prep the skin with antiseptic swab, using a circular motion
5. Insert needle into vein at a 10° angle using aseptic technique, and stabilizing the vein to prevent it from rolling
6. Aspirate to ensure entry and withdraw desired amount of blood
7. Release tourniquet
8. Withdraw needle, applying pressure to the site
9. Inject blood into tube(s)
10. Label tube(s) with patient information
11. Recheck puncture site for bleeding or hematoma
12. Report completion to hospital

Venipuncture Using Vacutainer
1. Gather necessary equipment
2. Attach Vacutainer needle to its holder
3. Insert Vacutainer tube into holder (avoid inserting needle into tube and breaking suction)
4. Identify appropriate site (usually antecubital fossa)
5. Apply constricting band proximal to site and distend vein
6. Prep skin with antiseptic swab, using a circular motion
7. Insert needle into vein at a 10° angle using aseptic technique and stabilizing vein to prevent it from rolling
8. Advance tube so needle pierces stopper; check for blood return
9. Allow tube to fill completely; change tubes as needed
10. Release tourniquet
11. Withdraw tube of blood from holder
12. Withdraw needle and apply pressure to site
13. Label tube(s) with patient information
14. Recheck puncture site for bleeding or hematoma
15. Report completion of procedure to hospital

SELF-ASSESSMENT QUESTIONS

Reference Pages

Antishock Trousers
337–338

1. Discuss the principles behind use of the antishock trousers in management of hypovolemic shock.

2. In which clinical conditions would antishock trousers be indicated?

3. Which conditions might be aggravated by application of the antishock trousers?

4. What is the one strict contraindication for use of the antishock trousers?

5. What are the landmarks for proper placement of the antishock trousers?

6. What are the sequential steps to follow when applying the antishock trousers?

7. What should be done if the patient complains of increasing respiratory difficulty or nausea/vomiting while the trousers are inflated?

8. When and by whom should the trousers be removed?

9. What complication can result if the antishock trousers are deflated suddenly?

Assessment
338–347

1. What are the components of the primary survey?

2. What elements are considered when assessing the scene?

3. What is included in assessment of the ABCs?

4. What consideration will be included in determining whether or not immediate transport is indicated?

5. What components are included in the secondary survey?

6. What is included in assessment of level of consciousness?

7. What is included in investigation of chief complaint?

8. What is included in gathering a pertinent medical history?

9. What components are included in assessment of vital signs, and what factors should be checked for each?

10. What elements are included in a rapid head-to-toe physical exam, and what factors are important in each?

11. How can the head-to-toe exam be modified to emphasize areas pertinent to the chief complaint?

12. How is assessment modified for children?

13. What are the differences between adult and pediatric vital signs?

14. How do you estimate a child's weight based on age?

15. When is re-assessment done and why is it necessary?

Auscultation of Chest Sounds   348—349

1. List indications for chest auscultation in the field.

2. What types of lung sounds can be auscultated?

3. Where are lung sounds best auscultated?

4. Discuss the implication of muffled heart sounds.

Cardioversion   349—350

1. List the indications for cardioversion.

2. List the accepted w/s settings used in cardioversion of a supraventricular tachycardia for a child and an adult.

3. What is the accepted w/s used in cardioversion of ventricular tachycardia?

4. What is the drug of choice for sedating a patient prior to cardioversion?

5. Define the purpose of synchronization in cardioversion.

6. What is the procedure used in cardioversion?

Communication Equipment Operation 350–352

1. List two alternative methods for communicating with the hospital and discuss when you would use each.

2. What does "line of sight" mean and how does it affect radio?

3. How might you augment your antenna?

4. List the steps necessary to communicate over the mobile radio.

5. How and when would you communicate using the telephone coupler?

6. What would you do if you could not establish communications with the hospital?

Communication Format 352–354

1. What information should be given in the initial radio transmission?

2. What additional patient information is reported in subsequent radio communications?

3. Why is it necessary to identify your unit with each transmission?

4. Why is it important to give a rapid synopsis of the situation?

5. How do you acknowledge a drug or treatment order?

Cricothyrotomy 354–356

1. Discuss the indications for cricothyrotomy.

2. Describe the location of the cricothyroid membrane.

3. List the steps followed in performing a cricothyrotomy by the
   a. incision method
   b. puncture method

4. What complications can occur following a cricothyrotomy and how can they be prevented?

Defibrillation 356–358

1. Define defibrillation.

2. What is the indication for defibrillation?

3. List the precautions employed while using a defibrillator.

4. What w/s setting is used to defibrillate an adult? A child?

5. How do you prepare the paddles for defibrillation?

6. Describe two acceptable sites of paddle placement for defibrillation.

7. List in proper sequence the steps taken prior to defibrillating a patient.

8. What two parameters should be assessed *immediately* after defibrillation?

9. What drug(s) might be ordered in conjunction with defibrillation?

EKG Monitoring and Telemetry   358–360

1. What types of patients require EKG monitoring?

2. What EKG monitoring lead(s) should be used in the field and why?

3. What skin preparation techniques should be performed to improve the EKG tracing?

4. What are the proper steps for sending an EKG via telemetry?

5. Why should you avoid unnecessary voice interruptions during the transmission of EKG to the hospital?

Endotracheal Intubation   360–361

1. Discuss the indications for endotracheal intubation.

2. Discuss the proper patient positioning for oral intubation for nasal intubation.

3. Describe the procedure of endotracheal intubation.

4. How is hyperoxygenation incorporated into the procedure?

5. How does one assure proper placement of the endotracheal tube?

6. List the complications that can occur during endotracheal intubation.

Esophageal Obturator Airway   362–363

1. When is an esophageal obturator airway indicated?

2. List the steps involved in the insertion of an EOA.

3. How much air is used to inflate the cuff of an EOA?

4. Discuss the precautions/contraindications for the use of an EOA.

5. What is the proper head and neck position for insertion of an EOA?

6. What complication(s) are associated with the EOA?

7. How do you check for proper placement of the EOA?

8. How do you assess the adequacy of ventilation with the EOA in place?

9. When should an EOA be removed in the field?

10. What phenomenon usually follows removal of an EOA, and what precautions should be taken?

Intracardiac Injections   363–365

1. When is an intracardiac (IC) injection indicated in the prehospital setting?

2. Name the medication(s) you are most likely to administer by the intracardiac route.

3. Give the anatomical landmarks for an IC injection in:
   a. an adult
   b. a child (3–12 years)
   c. an infant (newborn to 3 years)

4. Describe the technique(s) for administration of an IC injection to
   a. an adult
   b. a child (3–12 years)
   c. an infant (newborn to 3 years)

5. Why is aspiration necessary during advancement of the needle?

6. List the potential complications of an IC injection.

7. What can you do to assure that CPR is not interrupted any longer than absolutely necessary when you have been ordered to give an IC injection?

8. How would you determine the effectiveness of a medication given by the IC route?

Intramuscular and Subcutaneous Injections   365—366

1. When are IM injections given?

2. What sites can be used for IM injections in adults? In infants?

3. What is the proper needle size, angle of insertion, and technique for IM injections?

4. List medications that can be given by the IM route.

5. When are SC injections given?

6. What sites can be used for SC injections?

7. What is the proper needle size, angle of insertion and technique for SC injections?

8. List medications that can be given by the SC route.

9. Why is it necessary to aspirate before injecting any medication?

10. What are possible complications that could arise from IM or SC injections?

IV Insertion into the External Jugular Vein   367—368

1. What are the indications for an external jugular IV in the field?

2. How would you locate the external jugular vein?

3. List the methods for distending the external jugular vein.

4. List in sequence the steps involved in cannulating the external jugular vein.

5. Discuss the possible complications of an external jugular IV.

6. What should you do if bleeding or infiltration occurs around an external jugular IV?

7. How can you prevent a pneumothorax from occurring when inserting an external jugular IV?

IV Insertion into a Peripheral Vein   368—370

1. Discuss the reasons for starting a peripheral IV.

2. What are the types of needles/cannulas used for an IV initiation and when are they indicated?

3. Describe the criteria used for IV site selection.

4. How do you facilitate venous distension?

5. List the complications of IV therapy.

6. How do you keep the vein from rolling during venipuncture?

7. List signs that suggest that the IV has infiltrated.

8. What complications can occur if you place tape around the entire extremity in which an IV is running?

IV Insertion into the Subclavian Vein   370—371

1. When is a subclavian IV indicated?

2. What are the landmarks for the subclavian puncture?

3. List in sequence the proper steps in establishing a subclavian IV.

4. What are the possible complications following a subclavian cannulation.

5. List ways to prevent air embolism during subclavian cannulation.

6. What complication can occur if the cannula is moved around after insertion?

IV Medication Administration   371—374

1. List field situations in which medications may be ordered by the IV route.

2. List the four ways by which medications may be given intravenously.

3. Why is it important to make sure that you are in the vein when injecting a medication?

4. What should be reported to the hospital following administration of a

drug by IV route?

IV Set-Up   375–376

1. When do you use a microdrip? A maxidrip?

2. When do you use a Volutrol?

3. How can you determine that an IV solution is safe to use?

4. How far should the drip chamber be filled?

Magill Forceps   376–377

1. When are Magill forceps indicated?

2. Discuss precautionary measures when using the Magill forceps.

3. Discuss complications which can occur with the use of the laryngo-scope.

4. List in sequence the steps involved in removing an upper airway obstruction with the Magill forceps.

5. What support measures should be utilized during the procedure?

Nasogastric Intubation   377–378

1. What is the purpose of a nasogastric (NG) tube?

2. When might an NG tube be used in the prehospital setting?

3. How do you measure the length for proper placement of the NG tube?

4. List methods used to facilitate passage of an NG tube.

5. List in sequence the proper procedure for insertion of an NG tube.

6. List possible complication(s) from NG tube insertion.

7. If the patient coughs or cannot speak immediately following insertion of an NG tube, what has most likely occurred? What should you do to correct it?

8. How do you confirm proper placement of the NG tube?

9. What action is indicated when an NG tube becomes obstructed?

Pericardiocentesis   378–379

1. When is a pericardiocentesis indicated?

2. What are the signs indicating decreased cardiac output and a developing cardiac tamponade?

3. Describe in sequence the steps in performing pericardiocentesis.

4. What are the complications of pericardiocentesis?

5. What should you do if a puncture is unsuccessful?

Rotating Tourniquets   379–380

1. Give the indication for use of rotating tourniquets in the field.

2. What are the principles behind the use of rotating tourniquets?

3. How do you apply rotating tourniquets and what precautions should be used?

4. How often are the tourniquets rotated and in what sequence?

5. What complication can occur if all tourniquets are removed at once?

6. List other methods used in the field treatment of pulmonary edema.

7. What parameter(s) should be assessed to determine effectiveness of rotating tourniquets?

Suctioning   380–382

1. What is the purpose of suctioning?

2. List common field situations in which suctioning is indicated.

3. How would you modify your technique for:
   a. oropharyngeal suctioning
   b. deep tracheal suctioning

4. How do you position a conscious patient for tracheal suctioning? An unconscious patient?

5. How do you position a patient when using a tonsil tip pattern?

6. List in sequence the proper procedure for suctioning.

7. List in sequence the proper procedure for tonsil tip suctioning.

8. How do you determine when the suction catheter tip has reached the carina?

9. Why must high-flow oxygen be given before and after tracheal suctioning?

10. Discuss common complications of tracheal suctioning.

11. What parameter is used to assess the effectiveness of suctioning?

Thoracostomy (Needle)   382—383

1. When is a needle thoracostomy indicated?

2. List the signs and symptoms indicating a developing tension pneumothorax.

3. Give two acceptable sites where you may insert the needle to relieve a tension pneumothorax.

4. Describe the procedure for relieving a tension pneumothorax.

5. How do you know when the cannula has entered the pleural cavity?

6. What are complications which may occur when performing a needle thoracostomy?

Triage   383—386

1. What is the paramedic's role in a multiple casualty incident?

2. Who serves as triage officer, and what is the triage officer's role?

3. Where should the communications base be set up, and why?

4. What considerations are important to ensure clarity of communication?

5. What considerations are important to ensure accurate identification of patients?

6. What is triaging? How is it done? What categories are used, and what criteria determine assignment of patients to those categories?

7. What is included in the 30-second survey of each patient?

8. What is the restricted level of care appropriate to multiple casualty incidents?

9. How are patients assigned to ambulances for transport to hospitals?

Vagotonic Maneuvers 386–388

1. When are vagotonic maneuvers indicated?

2. Describe two types of vagal stimulation.

3. What precautions should be taken prior to vagal stimulation of any kind?

4. Describe the procedure for Valsalva's maneuver.

5. How does CSM work?

6. If carotid pulses are unequal which side would you massage?

7. Describe the procedure for CSM.

8. When should CSM be discontinued?

9. Discuss the dangerous side effects which can occur with vagal stimulation.

10. What action(s) should you take if CSM is ineffective?

Venipuncture 388–389

1. What is a venipuncture?

2. When are venipunctures performed in the field?

3. What is the main complication of a venipuncture?

4. What are the steps used to perform a venipuncture?
   a. using a needle and syringe
   b. using a Vacutainer

COMMON ABBREVIATIONS

Abbreviation	Meaning
$\bar{\text{a}}$	before
ABC	airway, breathing, circulation
ALS	advanced life support
AMI	acute myocardial infarction
amps	ampules
ANS	autonomic nervous systrem
ARP	absolute refractory period
ASA	aspirin
ASHD	arteriosclerotic heart disease
AT	atrial tachycardia
AV	atrioventricular
bicarb	sodium bicarbonate
BID	twice a day
BLS	basic life support
BP	blood pressure
BS	blood sugar
$\bar{\text{c}}$	with
Ca^+	calcium
$CaCl_2$	calcium chloride
CAD	coronary artery disease
CC	chief complaint
cc	cubic centimeter
CCU	coronary care unit
CHB	complete heart block
CHF	congestive heart failure
Cl^-	chloride
cm	centimeter
CNS	central nervous system
c/o	complains of
CO	carbon monoxide
CO_2	carbon dioxide
Code 3	respond as rapidly as possible, red light and siren
COPD	chronic obstructive pulmonary disease
CPR	cardiopulmonary resuscitation
CSF	cerebrospinal fluid
CSM	carotid sinus massage
CV	cardiovascular
CVA	cerebrovascular accident

Abbr	Meaning
D/C	discontinue
dig	digitalis
DOA	dead on arrival
DOE	dyspnea on exertion
DM	diabetes mellitus
D/W, D₅W, 5% D/W	5% dextrose in water
D₅₀W, 50% D/W	50% dextrose in water
Dx	diagnosis
EA, EOA	esophageal obturator airway
ED	emergency department
EKG, ECG	electrocardiogram
Epi	epinephrine
ER	emergency room
ET	endotracheal
ETOH	alcohol
fib	fibrillation
fl	fluid
fx	fracture
GI	gastrointestinal
gm	gram
gr	grain
gt(t)	drop(s)
h, hr	hour
HBD	has been drinking
hx	history
IC	intracardiac
ICU	intensive care unit
IM	intramuscular
IV	intravenous
K⁺	potassium
Kg	kilogram
KO	keep open
KVO	keep vein open
L	liter
LBB	left bundle branch
LOC	level of consciousness
μgtt	microdrops
MCl₁	modified chest lead, V₁
MD	doctor
mEq	milliequivalents
mg	milligram

Abbr	Meaning	Abbr	Meaning
MI	myocardial infarction	RBB	right bundle branch
MIC	mobile intensive care	RBC	red blood cell
MICN	mobile intensive care nurse	RHD	rheumatic heart disease
MICU	mobile intensive care unit	RL	Ringer's Lactate
min	minute	R/O	rule out
ml	milliliter	RN	registered nurse
mm	millimeter	RRP	relative refractory period
mv	millivolt	Rx	treatment
MS	morphine sulfate	s̄	without
+	sodium	SA	sinoatrial
Cl	sodium chloride	SC	subcutaneous
NaHCO₃	sodium bicarbonate	sec	second
G, N/G	nasogastric	SICU	surgical intensive care unit
nitro	nitroglycerine	SIDS	sudden infant death syndrome
NPO	nothing by mouth	SL	sublingual
NS	normal saline	SOB	shortness of breath
NSR	normal sinus rhythm	SPA	salt poor albumin
NTG	nitroglycerine	SQ	subcutaneous
O₂	oxygen	STAT	immediately
OB	obstetrics	s/s	signs/symptoms
OD	overdose	SVT	supraventricular tachycardia
OPP	organophosphate poisoning	Sx	symptoms
OR	operating room	TIA	transient ischemic attack
P	pulse	TID	three times a day
p̄	after	TKO	to keep open
PAC	premature atrial contraction	u.	unit
PAM	Protopam®	VF	ventricular fibrillation
PAT	paroxysmal atrial tachycardia	VS	vital signs
PE	physical exam, pulmonary edema	VT	ventricular tachycardia
pedi	pediatric	WAP	wandering atrial pacemaker
PERL	pupils equal, reactive to light	WBC	white blood cell
PJC	premature junctional contraction	w/s	watt/second setting
PNC	premature nodal contraction	x	times
PND	paraxysmal nocturnal dyspnea	y/o	years old
po	orally, by mouth		
PRI	P-R interval of EKG		
pr	per rectum		
prn	whenever necessary, as needed		
PVC	premature ventricular contraction		
q̄	every		
QID	four times a day		
R	respirations		

INDEX